The Other Side of Psychiatric Care

The 'New Approaches to Care' Series

Patients are people. They have feelings, families and fears. Whatever the cause for their seeking help, the caring professional will find that he or she will be concerned with these other issues. All illness carries with it anxiety and each person has very individual and important feelings about it; feelings which can easily be forgotten or neglected when nurses become preoccupied with the details of treatments, procedures and ward routines.

The 'New Approaches to Care' Series aims to explore this 'other side' of care in a practical and realistic way, emphasising the importance of meeting all the patients' needs, whilst recognising the constraints and problems which so often make the 'other side' the forgotten side of patient care.

The books in this series examine the implications that treatments, procedures, investigations and routines can have for patients and their families. They also aim to help nurses gain some insight into the problems, feelings and anxieties which people can experience when they are being looked after in hospital or the community. The series will thus offer a tangible starting point for all nurses and other professionals, both in training and in practice, to give their patients the most complete and understanding care possible.

Series Editors

June Jolly, SRN, RSCN has devoted most of her nursing career to the care of sick children, and was involved with establishing a new paediatric unit at Brook General Hospital, Woolwich.

Jill Macleod Clark, BSc, PhD, SRN is a Lecturer in the Department of Nursing Studies, Chelsea College, University of London.

Will Bridge, BSc, PhD is the Co-ordinator of the Learning Resources Unit at Brighton Polytechnic.

THE OTHER SIDE OF PSYCHIATRIC CARE

Margaret Garland, BA, RMN

Illustrated by Gillian Simmonds, ARCA

First published 1983 by
THE MACMILLAN PRESS LTD
London and Basingstoke
Companies and representatives throughout the world

Printed in Hong Kong

ISBN 0 333 33512 0 (hard cover)
     0 333 33513 9 (paper cover)

To Edwin Garland, my husband,
who drew my attention to this prayer
shortly before this book went to press:

'Oh, Great Spirit, help me never to
judge another until I have walked
two weeks in his moccasins.'

Sioux Indian Prayer

Contents

Preface

This book is one of a series which looks at the other side of caring for a range of *people* who — through no fault of their own — become *patients*.

The overriding purpose of the whole series, called *'New Approaches to Care'*, is to insist that patients are people, no matter what they may be suffering from, nor what their ages. The first book (June Jolly's *The Other Side of Paediatrics*) was about young patients and the second was about old patients (Pat Brown's *The Other Side of Growing Older*). So, if one thing comes over more than anything else, I hope it is the 'peopleness' of the psychiatric patients who appear in this book. It certainly is full of people: Stuart, Nancy, Shirley, Greg, Peter, right through to Pam, who is the last to be mentioned, though none is given his/her true name.

The importance — for all those who come into contact with psychiatric patients — of the interplay between person and person is highlighted in this book. 'Relationships' and 'interaction' are amongst the most common jargon words these days, but they are talked of so much because they are so important. So we have people, and people relating to each other, and one more special ingredient. In Chapter 1 I shall be emphasising my belief in the value of deliberately trying to step into the shoes of other people, and particularly those we care for, in order to consider how they may think and feel. I could have kept saying 'Imagine how that patient might feel when such and such happens'. Instead I have urged that we get closer: 'Let me imagine I am Stuart . . . Let me imagine I am Nancy. How do I feel?'

This book is to be about patients, psychiatric patients usually. It's for all those who care for them, starting from my viewpoint as a psychiatric ward sister, but relevant, I hope, to others who work in the psychiatric hospital, or in health care generally, or even those for whom the patient is their relative or friend. I want to show how helpful it is when patients, staff and relatives work together. So, as well as stepping into the shoes of the patients, we'll step also into the shoes of fellow staff, and the shoes of relatives.

I have included in a later chapter, specifically on the relatives of psychiatric patients, a description of 'the invaluable triangle' which encompasses psychiatric patients, staff and relatives. Although most of this book is about the patients, the chapters on the staff and the relatives are equally important.

As I have already said, it is the precise point of this series of books to recognise patients as people and to treat them as such. In our case, this involves looking at the sociological and psychological aspects of psychiatric care. But this is not to minimise the part that medical care must play in psychiatric care. The three are inextricably intertwined.

Chichester, 1982

M.G.

Acknowledgements

So very many people have contributed to the making of this book directly and indirectly, and I wish to thank them. This is, inevitably, far from a complete list.

Will Bridge, then a senior research officer of the Joint Board of Clinical Nursing Studies, and Jill Macleod Clark pioneered the *'New Approaches to Care'* Series, and invited me to write this. Will has guided me and kept my thoughts from straying too wildly. June Jolly, who had already written *The Other Side of Paediatrics*, and Elizabeth Horne, Macmillan's nursing editor, encouraged me. It was great to meet and to work with Gillian Simmonds, the artist, and I am much indebted to her for her contributions to this book.

But these people were not psychiatric experts. Reg Everest, director of nurse education at the Maudsley, read the first draft; and the final draft benefited from his comments. I showed a copy, too, to various nurses in my own hospital and to a tutor, Andy Bessant. All were so encouraging and helpful.

It may be considered remarkable that I sought the advice of so few of my present colleagues. That was because I knew I could only write this in my way. But very many have contributed to the way I think about psychiatric care and these are a few of their number.

Jim and Dora Warren helped train me and went on being available for me to talk to and listen to when I was a staff nurse and first a sister. Sister Garnett (I never called her anything else!) much influenced me during nine whole months of my training. Now I frequently wonder how she put up with me, when I see students being as impatient or as 'clever' or as 'wise' as I was. Margaret Storer, already a sister when I began to train, became a friend and a great listener and talker. I learnt about co-

counselling later, but Margaret and I co-counselled by instinct. Three consultants have played an important part in my career: Donald Dick, Tony Gumbrell and Norman Capstick. From the first I learnt to 'look for the normal rather than for the abnormal', from the second to consider the question 'What is schizophrenia?', and the third helped appoint me to my present sister's post where I have gone on listening and looking and talking and thinking and working things out and, as needed, adapting my views. My final thanks, therefore, to all who work with me, to the many patients I have come to know, and to their relatives, many of whom now feel like friends. God bless. We certainly are not islands.

Part One:

Patients as People

1 Patients First

Why We Must Start Here

Scene A sister's office in a mixed ward for patients who have been in hospital for some years. The sister and two student nurses are just about to sit down after the early activity of stirring the patients into getting up and going out of the ward for work or treatment. A conversation between the sister, a student and one of the patients has been of special interest, and the sister wants to talk it over.

Stuart arrives, in a bit of a rush, as so often. Slim and restless, he looks younger than might be expected at thirty.

Stuart (laughing) Yes, I know, Margaret! I am just going to work. But there's something I must say first.
Sister Are you sure, Stuart? I particularly wanted to talk to Nikki and Cathy at this moment.
Stuart It will be helpful to you nurses. Honestly, it will!
Sister OK, Stuart. Let's hear it!

Stuart settles down comfortably. Sister recognises that he is about to 'go on'. His opening words confirm her expectations.

Stuart Well, it's like this. They didn't teach me the facts of life in the army.
Sister Stuart! You'll get these two girls giggling! You don't really expect the army to teach the facts of life, do you?
Stuart No, that's not really what I mean. Look at it this way . . .

And he tries again. One has to give full marks to Stuart for persistence. And to the sister for helping him to spell it out. His first point, translated, emerges as something like: 'I know I am a young man with young ladies around me; yet I don't feel sexually aroused. I am wondering if the tranquillising injections, which I know I need, are also dampening my natural instincts.'

But he does not want that discussed at the moment. His main point is yet to come. And he gets that out clearly and simply.

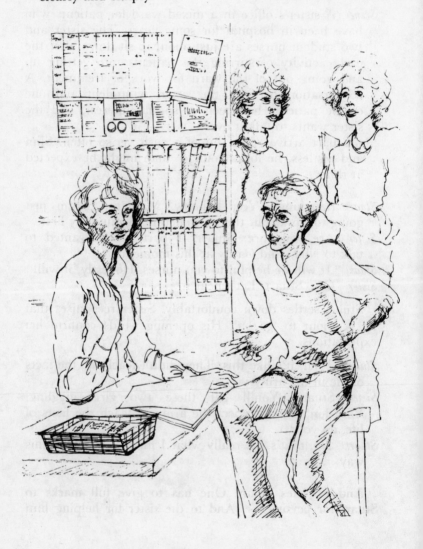

Stuart   You see, you don't discuss our real problems with us. You know, these people here sit around and worry a lot. They worry about themselves and how long they're going to be here and what's going to happen to them. They do, you know. I sit and watch them.

This conversation, like almost any with a patient, can provide several talking points. Let's single out this one: the sister wanted to discourage Stuart from talking then and, if he had not been persistent, the three nurses would not have heard a frank statement of his problems.

Stuart is not alone. In their own ways, and those ways are seldom as straightforward as Stuart's finally was, many psychiatric patients attempt to tell their nurses that they need more serious attention and help.

Do the patients come first in a psychiatric hospital? And if not, why not? The sole purpose of the hospital is for their benefit, but the nurses and other staff who work there frequently lose sight of this.

Where do patients fit in? And how does a psychiatric hospital tick in the 1980s? To answer the first we probably have also to answer the second. Once upon a time there was a hierarchical approach, staff-wise at least, with people knowing their position in the pecking order. It's not that I am totally opposed to a firm hierarchy - as a sister I know that, although we are now all equal on the ward, there are times when the sister needs to be 'more equal than others'. This is also to the others' benefit in that the sister will be prepared, at times, to accept the responsibility for their mistakes. But, given a pecking order, there is a danger that the patient will be below the lowest nurse and not above the highest consultant.

To draw a second point from the story of Stuart: at least he sees the sister as 'Margaret' and approachable. The multi-disciplinary system is much more in operation now, in theory anyway. And the patients, in theory, rank alongside the staff. Not ideal, maybe, but it is an improvement, isn't it?

This book is not a text-book. It does not concern itself

with varieties of psychiatric treatments. It is one nurse's attempt to discover what Stuart and his fellows feel, and an attempt to put across to the nurses, other health workers and friends of psychiatric patients our need to stay alert to *their* feelings.

2 Patients, Staff and Attitudes

Relationships - The Heart of the Matter

Let me start this chapter by paraphrasing a well known passage in the *Bible* (1 Cor. 13):

> I may be the most verbally able person imaginable,
>> but if I cannot relate comfortably to others,
>> it is in the end nothing but mere noise or words.
>
> I may be brilliant at seeing what lies ahead;
> I may have attended many courses, have many
>> qualifications, and have read many books;
> I may be a great achiever, a fantastic organiser,
>> but if I cannot relate comfortably to others,
>> I am useless.
> I may give all my money, my time, and indeed my whole
> life to my work,
>> but if I cannot relate comfortably to others,
>> in the end I cannot claim to have done anything at all.

THE NEED TO RELATE

From time to time Nancy talks about her damaged heart, especially on Fridays which are her washing-up days. 'Nancy is deluded again', we say. But read on. The following scene is not a Friday.

> *Nancy* . . . So could you get my sister to let me stay overnight with her regularly? Every week, unless of course she has something she really wants to go out for. You see, I do love my sister. We were very close once, but we've grown apart. I want to get closer to her again. I've had so much trouble over the years.

It's probably hard for you nurses to understand. I have this great pain in my heart. So much heartache now.

Sister (enlightened) Oh! Nancy, you quite often talk about having a damaged heart. I thought you meant you had a physically damaged heart. Do you mean you feel emotionally hurt?

Nancy Yes. I don't really have people to love me properly. And I want to get closer to my sister again.

The truth may be that Nancy sometimes gets muddled, because of her illness, into confusing her emotions and her physical state. Or the truth may be that Nancy has it right and we have it wrong - that emotional and physical states are even more closely linked than we realise. Let's leave all that. The point here is: people need people.

Is a need to relate comfortably to other people the key to the whole of psychiatry? Could one summarise it all like this:

Cause of the patient's illness	An inability to relate well to other people
Treatment	Helping the patient to relate
The cured patient	Lives outside the hospital, relating happily ever after to relatives, friends and workmates.

Let's look at how true this is, and how long we have known it. When Aristotle said 'Man is by nature a political animal', well over 2000 years ago, he was not talking about power struggles, but about man's need to live together in communities. Paul wrote urgently to friends in Corinth around the year A.D. 55 about the prime importance of relating comfortably to others (see my paraphrase at the start of this section), and John Donne spelled out in the 1600s that 'No man is an island'. It is not a new idea. The tragedy is that we in the 1980s may quote the words of

Paul and Donne as beautiful literature and not apply the meaning to the way we live. So we need to restate that people need to relate well to others. John Powell (1969) has done so in *Why Am I Afraid to Love?* and *Why Am I Afraid to Tell You Who I Am?* People's need for people is frequently the theme of novels, poems and pop songs.

So, the need to relate comfortably may have to be spelled out again and again. But then we have to ask and to answer, '*How* do we learn to relate comfortably to others?'

Perhaps we can see psychiatric nursing like a football match. Good relationships are the goals. There will be much tackling on the way to the goals, and wrong moves and penalties. But there will also be trainers and coaching sessions, and there can be first class teamwork.

'ME-ME-ME!'

If the breakdown of relationships is a key feature of mental illness, isn't the self-centredness of the mentally ill the other side of the same coin?

Just listen to the patients: 'Can I have? . . . I want . . . Why can't I?' Think around the different faces of mental illness and consider what such patients are saying. The depressed patient, the hypochondriacal, the anxious, the phobic: 'I really can't be bothered . . . I'm worried about my . . . I don't think I'd be able to manage that . . . I have this awful fear.' The manic - we had to ease one out of our last ward party; she had drifted in from an acute ward and had discovered our piano. Yes, she could play and sing very well, but we had never even seen her before, and this was about to become her party! Look at the withdrawn schizophrenic and the bizarre: they are in their own worlds, not ours.

Psychiatric nurses have to look hard at their own feelings about the patients' self-centredness. The very new and keen nurse does not notice it; everything is novel and interesting and there is so much to take in. But after a while she begins to exclaim in astonishment, 'Isn't Ann selfish!' And a nurse who has been there longer may reply with some cynicism, 'They are all incredibly selfish!'

The leader of a caring community was visiting a psychiatric hospital and was extremely impressed by the patients he was meeting. 'Why ever are they here?' he asked the consultant, 'They can talk so sensibly!' 'Indeed they can,' the consultant replied, 'but mostly about themselves.'

We cannot ignore this characteristic. And we must come to terms with it or we shall tend to feel, though probably not express it, 'These patients are not worth bothering about.'

Sometimes we may actually express it.

Scene   The ward's large sitting room is occupied by nine people sitting in a circle - a consultant, two registrars, the sister, a community psychiatric sister, the social worker, two student nurses and one patient, who may have to come back into hospital.

Consultant   Your landlady and fellow tenants are complaining because you play records loudly through the night.

Patient (smiling)   That's right.

Consultant   And expect breakfast when you get up at 2 p.m.

Patient (smiling)   Yes.

Consultant   Why do you do it?

Patient   I like playing records at night, but then I'm too tired to get up early.

Consultant   Don't you think that is a little hard on the other people who live there?

Patient   I suppose so.

Consultant   Could you not possibly change that habit?

Patient   I don't know. Not very easily.

The ward sister is tired and human and has become intolerant. She looks around the circle and estimates the salaries of those who are bringing their minds to bear on this problem.

Sister (after the meeting to the social worker) Oh,
honestly! I was watching that programme about lions
last night. If Jack were a gazelle he'd have dropped
behind and been gobbled up long ago! Oh, I
shouldn't say such things, I know!
Social worker (giving her a friendly hug and laughing)
I know how you feel! We all feel like that sometimes.
Never mind. Cheer up; you've got your holiday next
week, haven't you!

We shall look later at the abundance of causes of stress
in psychiatric hospital staff. Here we can record that one
cause is the wear and tear of patients' self-centredness.

While accepting that it is human to find this stressful at
times, we must keep reminding ourselves of these three
points:

Being turned in on oneself is part of an inability to
relate well to other people.
The inability to relate well to other people is a
severe handicap to normal living.
Helping people to relate to others is at the heart of
our work.

Staff-Patient Attitudes

GETTING ATTITUDES RIGHT

Point one of this book has now been spelled out: Forming
good relationships is at the heart of mental health. Point
two: Unless the staff's attitudes to the patients are good,
the patients cannot learn to form relationships.

And, alas, isn't it an area in which we do not readily
change either ourselves or others? We all believe our
attitudes are already right!

'I am firm and she is soft.'

'I am kind and she is harsh.'

We so readily justify our attitudes. Take 'teasing' as a
single example. 'I am only teasing!' I say when I've said

something mischievous to a patient I think I know very well and have then wondered if I've gone too far and hurt his feelings. 'We only tease the people we like!' we used to tell Helen, a very distraught young lonely woman who in the end recognised and accepted our liking for her that permitted us to tease her gently. And yet 'We were only teasing!' I've heard nurses say in justification of some mickey-taking that to my mind was near to mental cruelty.

Nurses with good attitudes, especially students who are circulating and meeting a lot of different nurses, sometimes need reassurance that what they feel to be right is right. The authoritative nurse so often gets immediate obedience from a patient who is being uncooperative. 'See! I have no trouble with him!' can be very demoralising to someone who is still learning and not yet certain of her own approach.

My paraphrase at the start of the passage on relationships was first written in a moment of bitterness with the non-relating nurses in mind.

If we listen we shall find that the patients do tell us what they think of our attitudes.

> *Scene*   A ward dormitory. Sister is talking to a patient, Jean.
>
> *Sister*   Some of the patients do act a bit madly sometimes. And the staff.
> *Shirley*   (from behind her bed-curtains) Especially the staff.

On her way out of the dormitory the sister sits on Shirley's bed with her. She had been transferred to the ward a week earlier and had done little but sit lumpily and glower. When asked, she confirmed that she did not feel happy but would say no more.

> *Sister*   The nurses do ass about sometimes, don't they, Shirley!
> *Shirley*   It's not that. They treat us as if they own us. And they don't.

Sister I do try to get it right, Shirley, and I know I often
fail. Keep on helping us. Point out when we get it
wrong.

Shirley No, we can't do that. The nurses don't like it
when we do that.

Later, the sister recounts with pleasure the way that
Shirley has spoken up. Only then does it occur to her to
wonder if anyone properly explained to Shirley why she
was being transferred. She arrived on a day when
everything was happening. On reflection, Shirley had
actually been looking like a heavy parcel that has been
lugged from place to place.

Patients will tell us if we listen, I said. Is that completely
true? In the passage about Shirley notice first how she
spoke from behind her curtains. Was she sure that she
would even be heard? She only said three words. Unlike
Stuart who began this book, Shirley is not persistent. In
Shirley's case it was the sister who had to persist to get at
the very strong feelings that Shirley held.

This whole section is chiefly concerned with the
attitudes of the staff to the patients. Relating well to other
people in fact is a two-way process. The ideal is that both
the attitudes of the staff to the patients and the attitudes of
the patients to the staff will become healthy enough for
good relationships to form. But while relating to others is a
problem for patients, often the initiatives will have to come
from the staff. 'Behaviour therapy' is a term that is now
used in a specialised way. But we control one another's
behaviour all the time by the way we approach one
another. A good nurse-patient attitude will help a patient
to relate to the nurse; a poor attitude will turn the patient
away - and an attitude that the patient feels to be
threatening may lead him to attack the nurse!

Here is a second, and happy, comment from a patient to
a nurse about her attitude.

Scene The staff nurse is new to the ward. She is a
cheerful friendly young lady who has already shown

that she is prepared to give the patients a great deal of time, and she has initiated many new activities.

Greg I am bored. Isn't there anything I can do?

Nurse Greg! All the things I ask you to do and you won't! Oh, you make me feel so cross! You really do! Whatever are we going to do with you, eh?

Peter (who is very much a loner, chirpily teases the nurse as he passes) Ah, you're getting snappy too now, aren't you!

The staff nurse passes on that comment to her fellow nurses both wrily, acknowledging that Peter's comment is true, and also with pleasure that he has been able to comment and that his attitude to her was so good while making the comment.

But wasn't he responding to her overall attitude? She had been a good model, as it were, that he was able to copy.

We have had three examples now of patients criticising nurses: Stuart maintaining that the nurses did not talk with the patients about their real problems; Shirley saying that the nurses treated patients as if they owned them; and Peter joking to the staff nurse about her snappiness.

There will be times when the patient's behaviour to the nurse is very much more aggressive, verbally or physically. What is to be the attitude of the nurse then?

Nurses who have found themselves in frightening situations may laugh cynically and say that there will be no time then to consider one's attitude. 'Act first and think later' may seem to be necessary.

Two points: first, that when the staff attitudes to the patients are good, there is much less disturbed behaviour; secondly, if the nurse's attitude is usually right, the nurse's instinctive reaction at a moment of danger is likely to be right too. My own most endangered moment to date was when I was in a small single room with a large strapping patient, Mary. A manic depressive, she was beginning to come out of an extremely low period. I was encouraging her to get up and she was reluctant. One arm was already into her dressing gown and I was helping her thread her second arm in when I saw her fist swinging upwards fast towards my face. Through my mind flashed 'Help! This is it! And I'm alone!' What I actually said was 'Mary!' and her hand went down. Why? Did I convey in that use of her name and in my surprised reproachful tone that this was not the sort of behaviour I expected from her? That she could be reasonable? That our relationship was usually good? Did the use of her name remind her that she was not only a person to me, but Mary, a particular person and friend?

ARE PATIENTS PEOPLE?

Let me try another paraphrase, this time of Shakespeare's *Merchant of Venice*:

> I am a patient. Hath not a patient eyes? Hath not a patient hands, organs, dimensions, senses, affections, passions? Fed with the same food, hurt with the same weapons, subject to the same diseases, healed by the same means, warmed and cooled by the same winter and summer, as a nurse is? If you prick us, do we not bleed? If you tickle us, do we not laugh? If you poison us, do we not die?

The attitudes of nurses and other staff to patients will encourage, or will discourage, the patients' ability to relate to them (and, ultimately, to other people - but that is a point to which we shall work bit by bit).

We must now ask how the staff see the patients? First and foremost, do we all see them as people? A distressed student nurse once brought to my attention that one of her fellow nurses had said to a patient, 'You are nothing but an animal!' Another student nurse had heard some non-nursing hospital workers who did not come much into contact with the patients say, 'Well, of course, they don't really feel pain like we do, do they?' These are viewpoints I find completely astounding and I record them merely to alert others to their existence, however rare now.

Yet, how rare is the attitude that psychiatric patients are somehow not quite as human as other people are? All psychiatric nurses are familiar with the statement 'Oh, I do admire you! I couldn't do your work!' The implication is that we are dealing with beings who are not like ourselves.

Patients are people. The very fact that we need to repeat that statement shows that even nurses who believe themselves to be dedicated professionals may be getting the emphasis wrong. In general nursing they may look at 'the appendix next to the window'. In psychiatric nursing we may see 'that schizophrenic' . . . 'that agoraphobic' . . . 'that psychopath' . . . 'that anorexic'. So much attention is being directed at seeing the whole patient and not the part now, that little by little our view of the patient is probably changing. But it does need to change and this book is directed towards changing it.

The very new and keen nurse mentioned earlier probably does see the patient as a person! A frequent question from students in their preliminary training weeks when they visit a ward is 'Why ever is Beryl here? She seems so normal!' The truth is that Ann and Beryl and Cynthia and Derek and Ernest and Felicity and George and all the patients are very normal people, very like the staff, in very many ways.

Of all I was ever taught, this made the greatest impact: 'We must stop looking for the patients' abnormalities and must recognise all their normal behaviour.' I do not believe the consultant who tossed off that comment in an on-the-ward discussion realised the impact it might make on any of his listeners. I am certain that he himself had looked for and recognised the normal behaviour of his patients for so long that it had become his completely natural approach.

But we student nurses were by then busy learning about disorientation, delusions, memory loss, hallucinations, thought disorder, and much more. Over meals we swopped stories of 'lunatic' behaviour to the point of one-upmanship.

'Alice climbed out of the window again today. She totters round the ward looking like a Parkinson, and then she hares off down the road in her nightie as fast as an Olympic sprinter!'

'We had a new admission today who says he has an eye in his leg and that people talk to him through it!'

From that beginning I too developed the habit of looking for and recognising the normal behaviour in all the patients on every ward until this has now become my automatic approach. I tend to assume it is the approach of other nurses, and it *is* the approach of very many nurses. But I am still reminded that it is not universal, by conversations I overhear in which abnormal behaviour is being delightedly reported.

However, here are three reasons for not swinging to the extreme of believing that the patients are wholly normal. It *is* necessary for students to learn to recognise factors such as delusions and hallucinations. It *is* necessary for us to recognise the patients' abnormalities in order that we shall have a better chance to know what help the patient needs. And, at the extreme, it may be dangerous not to recognise a patient's increasing distress.

Peter nearly strangled a nurse one evening. It was the worst attack I have been close to in my eight years in psychiatric nursing and it was extremely distressing for everyone: for the nurse, very obviously, but equally distressing for Peter himself, for the staff, and for Peter's fellow patients.

Analysing this situation is a good moment to introduce the idea of 'the golden mean'. It is a literal translation of a Roman phrase, *aurea mediocritas,* but the Greeks also had words for it: 'nothing to excess'. Keeping a middle course between two extremes is frequently wise. Here it applies to getting the right balance between seeing the psychiatric patient as exactly like ourselves, wholly normal (whatever that may mean!), and seeing the patient as wholly strange, mad, lunatic, frightening, psychotic, or whatever word one might choose.

The next example shows the wrongness of expecting totally normal behaviour from a patient who had been 40 years in a psychiatric hospital. A student nurse who had escorted Maggy on the pantomime-and-tea outing so generously arranged by the League of Friends speaks first:

Nurse   Oh I must tell you what Maggy did before you hear about it from Nora. It was awful! Maggy loved the pantomime but at teatime one of the League of Friends' ladies was fussing over her and Maggy smacked her face. I apologised and said that Maggy was enjoying herself very much in her quiet way but got very upset if she felt fussed. The woman said, 'My dear girl, I wasn't fussing her!' in a hoity-toity voice, and she went back to Maggy - and Maggy smacked her face again!

Now the comments of Nora, an older woman who had recently become an occupational therapy aide. Nora's attitude to the patients within the hospital was warm and helpful and she came across initially as someone who recognised the patients' normality. But she had not learnt also to accept their abnormality.

Nora   It was terrible! I'll never go out with the patients again. That poor woman! What a way to be treated - and when the League of Friends had put on such a marvellous time for the patients, too! How can the nurses send patients on outings who don't know how to behave!

But it was a good League of Friends and, although that particular League of Friends' helper had to learn, uncomfortably, more about the way to approach a patient, most of the helpers were better experienced and took mishaps in their stride.

So, let's repeat the need for the golden mean. Ideally the nurses and other staff will recognise that the patients are generally people who are very like themselves, but they will also make allowances for the abnormalities due to the patient's illness or inexperience in handling situations.

How normal are the patients? 'They are 90% normal, aren't they!' I said excitedly to a tutor in the early days of my nurse training. '95%!' he replied. It will vary from patient to patient and from situation to situation. Subjected to stresses, patients may quickly reveal their abnormalities. Nevertheless I still maintain that being treated as normal very much helps them towards normal behaviour.

> *Scene* The ward office. Nancy, who is often very suspicious, has taken to getting the ward staff to keep her purse in the office desk. The charge nurse has just given it to her, but she is standing in the office, peering into the purse and frowning ominously. The charge nurse wonders for a moment how best to tackle the unspoken accusation.

> *Charge nurse* Look here, Nancy, what is the point of giving that purse to us to look after if you think we are going to take your money out of it. I can assure you there is still exactly the same amount in it as when you last gave it to us!
> *Nancy* Oh yes, of course! Thank you! (And Nancy cheers up and goes off brightly.)

It would have been so easy to reason 'Poor Nancy. This is typical of her paranoid schizophrenia. I must handle her cautiously.' Instead he allowed himself to try out what he felt as an ordinary person, and on this occasion it reassured her and produced a more reasonable, a more 'normal' reaction from the patient.

ARE PATIENTS ILL?

We have now established, I hope, that patients can be seen as 'normal' much of the time, if the nurses are prepared to look for their normal behaviour and their normal comments. I would, personally, like to maintain the perhaps naive claim of my early student nurse days that patients may be normal 90% of the time. And that even the most bizarre and most disturbed have feelings very similar to our own, as we can see if only we are prepared to consider them.

Now for a gigantic question: 'Is "ill" the right word for these people?'

Let's look at people with physical problems. Is a one-legged man 'ill'? Are blind people 'ill'? The man who was in intensive care last year following a heart attack and who now regularly takes his tablets, is he still 'ill'?

A fair proportion of the people who read this book will be called 'psychiatric nurses' and work in 'hospitals'. These places were not always hospitals. Nurses are quite likely to be working in the 'asylum' that was built in the mid-nineteenth century, and which was then staffed by 'attendants' and headed by 'medical superintendents'.

What's in a name? A word is a word is a word. 'A rose by any other name would smell as sweet.' But that's not really true, is it? Words have associations. Say 'rose' and a picture comes into one's mind of a beautifully formed flower, petal within petal, with an almost indescribable sheen on those petals, and a wonderful colour and a heavenly scent.

'Asylum' means 'a place of refuge'. But the picture that began to form when people used that word was of a frightening place to which people were sent when they went out of their minds, where they remained in a state of insanity, from which they occasionally escaped, and from which they seldom returned into normal society. 'Hospital' was an improvement. It was far more acceptable to think of one's relative as 'ill', under the care of 'doctors' and 'nurses' who would work out what the 'patient' was 'suffering from' and 'prescribe suitable medicines' or other 'courses of treatment'.

Recently we have begun to look again at these words and to question the 'medical model'.

Scene   The corridor of a psychiatric hospital. A sister and her ward's consultant are about to pass.

Sister   Did you see Celia this morning? She's heaps better. It's nice, isn't it!

Doctor It is nice. But are you sure 'better' is the right word?

Sister (grinning) Go on, explain.

Doctor If we say Celia is 'better' now, aren't we suggesting that she has been 'ill'?

Sister (really puzzled now) But she's still very ill, isn't she?

Doctor If you say someone is 'ill', doesn't that imply you are looking for a 'cure'? And are we ever going to cure Celia? Isn't it rather that Celia has problems that she will have to learn to live with?

Sister (making a mental leap as the sight and sound of Celia comes into her mind) Oh - and Celia herself does not even see herself as 'ill'. Whenever I say, 'You're much better these days, Celia, aren't you!', she gets quite angry and says, 'I've not done anything wrong. I don't know what you're all on about.' I never understood her reaction. But we've been using 'better' differently, haven't we!

One could make a claim for now dropping 'hospital'. One could even make a claim for reverting to 'asylum' in its original sense, a place of refuge. Many of our patients appear to need a place of refuge to which they can withdraw for a while to give themselves a breathing space while they come to terms with the problems and pressures of their everyday lives.

A large book might deal with the medical *v* social models of psychiatric care, and with the precise nature of a patient's malady. A summary here: The 'golden mean' almost certainly applies. In some cases there appears to be a physical malfunction, that is, an 'illness', and in other cases an environmental or circumstantial cause, that is, a 'problem'. Often there is a mixture. It frequently appears to be very difficult indeed to determine the extent to which a psychiatric patient suffers from a physical illness and the extent to which it is a social problem. We shall look at this in more depth in Chapter 4.

The chief point of this section is: Please let us *not* take it for granted that every patient is to be considered to be 'ill'.

HOW DO NURSES SEE THEIR ROLE?

If all patients are normal much of the time, and if some of them should never properly be described as 'ill', how do nurses and others in the caring professions see their roles? A good question, I think. But I have no very simple answer.

Historically psychiatric nurses have been 'attendants'. They have also been seen as 'custodians'. One Women's Institute secretary welcoming patients from the ward where I was a student nurse had written, 'We shall be glad to have two or three of your patients at our meetings, provided they have an escort.' Edna, Doris, Sue and I all looked much alike - and much like the W.I. members themselves - and I amused myself during the evening by watching our hosts play 'spot the escort'. At the end of the meeting they were still not certain who was who, though they did not like to say so. The four of us had all behaved impeccably and had all joined in conversations quite normally. On that occasion we had all played a 'Women's Institute member' role.

There will still be times when a nurse has to be a custodian, especially on an admission ward when a new patient is acutely disturbed. For one reason or another such patients may not want to stay. They may have no insight into their need for help, or they may have more insight than we realise, but be terrified of the unknown place, fellow patients, and what may be done to them. It will be necessary sometimes for the nurse to convey 'I am sorry, but for the present you do need to stay here and we must keep you.' The nurse is then making clear, either in such words or by her actions, that she is a custodian.

Let us look a little further at the nurses who are initially in a custodial role. They will be able to play a befriending role at the same time. A special sympathy and an excellent relationship often develops between patients and the nurses who have helped them through a crisis. And the role may be subtly changing all the time from the decisive custodian, through the persuasive adviser, gentle encourager, to the relaxed companion and laughing friend. And even back to the start and through the progression again - oh, the embarrassment for a nurse, usually early in training, who has been lulled into becoming too relaxed too soon! (Question: should a nurse so inexperienced be left with a patient in need of custodial care? Answer (another question!): can a nurse properly learn the need to stay alert, without discovering the importance of alertness through experience?)

But what other roles may a psychiatric nurse be called upon to play alongside the patient? - sister, brother, mother, father, wife, husband, daughter, son, teacher, learner, . . . sometimes 'nurse' to a physically sick patient.

The need for the psychiatric nurse to have a variety of roles at his or her disposal is gradually becoming better understood. I copied this out in 1973 because it was what I was then finding for myself:

> Three or four young student nurses said that they would prefer to work on the sick ward - 'That's the only place in a mental hospital where you do proper nursing.' The point seemed to be that 'proper nursing' involved what might be called the technical trappings of the nursing profession - masks and white coats, oxygen cylinders and sterilisers, all the things which make up an adolescent's dream of what it means to be a nurse. (Jones and Sidebotham, 1962)

It is now much better recognised that looking after the sick is only one very tiny part of psychiatric nursing, and thankfully, it has now even been found that psychiatric patients with physical illnesses can almost invariably be nursed in the general hospital, looking and truly being quite normal! And how many psychiatric nurses have found during their weeks gaining physical nursing experience in the general hospital that many 'normal' people have been, temporarily at least, more psychiatrically disturbed than the patients in their own hospital!

A word of caution! The golden mean applies again as we consider our roles.

At one extreme we need to be conscious that we do assume various roles whether we are realising it or not. Are we, in fact, in some sort of role whenever we are with another person, and sometimes (always, perhaps) even when we are alone? That needs a lot more thought, but not now. For the moment, please accept this: we need to be aware from time to time of the role we are playing.

At the other extreme we can probably overdo our awareness of roles. We are likely to appear artificial if we are all the time thinking 'What role is needed at this moment? What role am I actually playing now?'

Ideally those who care for psychiatric patients should be chameleons, changing instinctively to suit the moment without taking thought. Could there be chameleons that ask themselves, 'Where am I now? Oh, against a red brick wall. I must change to "red brick".' I don't see them as great survivors, somehow, if it has to be such a conscious effort.

So, while initially the nurses may have to become aware of the playing of roles, better the nurses who get it wrong occasionally, when at least they will be recognised as 'human', than the very self-conscious nurse who tries to get it right all the time and who appears like an automaton.

WHAT ROLE IS THE PATIENT TO PLAY?

It seems from my own experience - and over my 50 years I have been many things, an introverted only child, a mixed-up schoolteacher and a happy mother - that we are often what people imagine us to be. Treated as stupid we are ham-handed and bungling. Treated as dull we are bores. But treated as bright we sparkle, and treated (as hopefully we all are at least sometimes in our lives) as the most wonderful person in the world, we are absolutely radiant!

Our patients will to a large extent play whatever role we cast them in. Treat them as normal and they become more normal. Treat them as patients and they are likely to play the patient role.

OK, next question: what is a patient role? Not just in a psychiatric hospital but anywhere.

Isn't it changing? Aren't patients generally being encouraged to speak up for themselves, to be co-workers with the doctors and nurses in the attempt to sort out their illness? In a speech to the 1980 cancer nursing conference, Mara Flaherty, a cancer patient, spelled out the need she had had over 14 years to work alongside the doctors and nurses (Flaherty, 1981).

Many patients always have taken that attitude, both as physically and as mentally ill people. But the patient picture is still perhaps of a person who goes to the doctor, asks for help, dutifully and unquestioningly obeys the instructions that are given, says 'Thank you, doctor' and 'Thank you, nurse', is neat and tidy and worked on, nicely submissive until cured and discharged from our scene to other roles in the big, wide world.

It is being recognised that 'ill' may not be the best description of many psychiatric patients anyway, and some, like Celia mentioned in the doctor-sister conversation, may not see themselves in an 'ill' role. But very many will. It is an acceptable role both to the patients, and to their families, and also to those of us who call ourselves 'nurses'!

If these people were still termed 'lunatics', would there be so many residents? What a question! And really it is too complex to answer. These pages are trying to say that the term, the roles and the attitudes are inextricably bound up. Call them 'lunatics' and the staff will treat them as lunatics and they will behave as lunatics. But would perhaps fewer people be prepared to accept the lunatic label than are now prepared to accept the psychiatric patient label?

However, the point of this section is to alert ourselves to the danger of these people seeing themselves as psychiatric patients, of adopting an 'I am ill and happy to put myself in your hands' role.

Aren't psychiatric nurses often very two-faced? There is a tendency to cast these people in a patient role first, insisting that they need our help, and then become cross with them when they go on playing that role beyond the time that we decide is reasonable?

THE ADULT-ADULT APPROACH

The full meaning of adult-adult relationships only occurred to me when I read a fascinating book by Eric Berne and came to grips with the idea of transactional analysis and *Games People Play* (Berne, 1966). Transactional analysis looks at the way that people adopt a 'parent', 'adult' or 'child' approach towards their relationships with each other. In an adult-adult approach each treats the other as a reasonable being on an equal footing.

Let me recap. We aim as psychiatric nurses to help our patients to relate comfortably to other people. Our attitude to them, how we see our patients, and how they see themselves will all help them towards the goal of good relationships, or if these are wrong will drive them away from that goal.

Can one have an adult-adult relationship, in which one looks at people as reasonable beings, if they are not appearing like reasonable beings? I have answered that already: how patients appear will depend very largely on what we are looking for. We should be looking for the very great deal of normal behaviour that is there and which we shall see only if we are looking and only if we are prepared to see it.

Yes, I will be honest. I have already said, also, that there is a great deal of wear and tear on people in the position of psychiatric nurses, and it would be unjust not to recognise this. The patients do have relationship difficulties, they are very wrapped up in themselves, and they do not manage to behave in a socially acceptable way the whole time; that is why they are under the care of the psychiatric team. There will be times when, however great our wish to see the patients' normal behaviour, it is their abnormal behaviour which intrudes upon us!

Nevertheless, I have found nothing so rewarding as getting normal responses from patients in return for the normal approaches I make.

Scene   7.15 a.m. in the dormitory.

Me   Good morning, Nancy . . . Good morning, Cindy . . . Good morning, Shirley (with a little bit more chat at some beds) . . . Good morning, Sheila.
Sheila   Good morning, Margaret.

That last word meant so much! She normally called me 'Sister'.

I am refusing to take part in any debate as to 'should the ward sister be called Margaret?' Maybe that will be a question that others still wish to ask. I don't. I am prepared to be 'Margaret' to anyone who is prepared to call me that. I am aware that some can not, and that at the extreme they call me 'Sister'. (None is so extreme as to call me 'Sister Garland'!)

Some adopt a half-way stance and call me 'Sister Margaret'. I am so used to this that I no longer even notice the oddity of it, though new students, doctors and visitors grin and sometimes use it mischievously themselves! But I remember, with pleasure and mischievousness on my own side, when I was shopping with Pauline, a very awkward young lady who normally uses 'Sister' as a clear barrier. We were buying wool together and in the middle of a sentence she had committed herself to calling me something. We both saw her mind work; which was it to be - 'Sister' or 'Margaret'? 'Margaret' and we grinned at each other. 'My round', as it were. Just for then though, in the normal surroundings; in the hospital, I am still 'Sister'.

Does that all sound like a mountain out of a molehill? It is out of such small matters that all those who care for psychiatric patients can get joy from their job, and from such small starts that patients can progress towards better relationships.

It will take time. The people most recently added to the psychiatric consultant's case-list have not developed their problems overnight. Even if, to a spectator, the onset has been sudden, it will in fact have taken time for them to reach this stage. And it will take some time to correct the problems. So what of the patients who have lived with their problems in psychiatric hospitals for many, many years? The people who are not involved in psychiatry boggle again and again when they hear the answers.

The longest resident I knew had been born in a workhouse around the turn of the century and, so the story went, been transferred to the asylum after cheeking the workhouse master. The truth of Alf's history was difficult to determine after so many years. In fact he did have a very good relationship with the hospital's staff by the time our group of student nurses first met him as our practice patient for hospital examinations. But between Alf with three-quarters of a century in institutions and the newest admission on the acute ward were hundreds of other patients with many years in the hospital. Again and again, in different ways, one became aware of it. One student nurse found coins with the year of Mary's admission: pre-decimal coins with the head of George V. Chance brought to my notice that Maureen, whom I had known to be about my own age and with whom I had built a happy relationship despite her continuing almost entirely silent, had come into hospital in exactly the same week as I had first met my husband. What a world of difference there had been in our two lives over all those years!

I record all that to make this one point: do not be surprised if you do not get a totally normal response the first time you behave normally towards a psychiatric patient. But do not give up.

In another book about transactional analysis, *I'm OK - You're OK*, Harris (1973) quotes from an article by Hailberg:

Treatment begins with the first exchange of glances between the therapist and patient, when the therapist enters with the basic position I'M OK - YOU'RE OK. Psychotics are yearning to establish a more meaningful relationship with people. When these usually very perceptive individuals are confronted by an individual who assumes the position I'M OK - YOU'RE OK this is a new and intriguing experience for them.

I leapt about with excitement when I read that. It confirmed what I had been finding for myself.

We see what we expect to see. Expect to see 'withdrawn schizophrenics' and you will see withdrawn schizophrenics. I had seen withdrawn schizophrenics. And yet? So often I had the impression that they were not withdrawn wholly from choice; that they were peeping at life from the sidelines and would have liked to have joined in if only they dared, if only they knew how, and if only they had persistent encouragement.

All along I used that expression, 'peeping at life from the sidelines', to myself about the withdrawn patients. Later I was given the idea of the aim of psychiatry being the goal of good relationships. The two went together and the football analogy I used earlier emerged!

Turning the psychiatric patient into a fully active participant in life - turning a non-sporting person with two left feet and the conviction that he will be no good at the game, and who is pretty sure most of the time that he does not want to join in anyway, into an eager and good footballer - won't be easy!

There will have to be a lot of individual, one-to-one, coaching. But first of all the spectator must be approached with an honest and friendly invitation: 'Come on, join us! We want you in on this!'

This is what an adult-adult approach does.

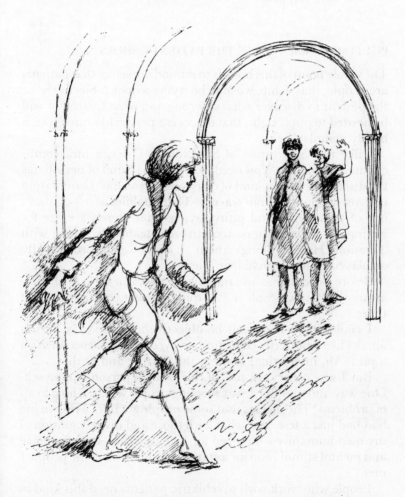

Scene The nurses are going off at the end of the day. Liz, a strange soul, is doing her usual odd little ritual of a dance in the ward's corridor near the office. Often

when approached Liz shouts 'Go away! Go away!' But
every night the nurses include Liz in the farewells.
Goodnight, Mary . . . Goodnight, Betty . . . Goodnight,
Liz. See you in the morning.' This night Liz stops her
dance, looks at the nurses and smiles: 'Goodnight!'
she says happily.

PUTTING OURSELVES IN THE PATIENTS' SHOES

The whole point of this book is to remind ourselves that patients
are people; that, while we may be trying to look 'objectively' at
the patient to discover what is wrong and what treatment will
be needed to put it right, that object is a person like ourselves, a
highly complex being.

I like the exhortation of Sir William Osler, a nineteenth-
century physician: 'You need to know what kind of person has
the disease, not what kind of disease a person has' (a quotation
in a nursing journal, not traced). That qualifies as a 'pot-shot',
one of those witty and pithy sayings that there's a craze for
having on cards, posters, teeshirts and teatowels. Along with
'Caution - Human Beings About', it could well be prominently
displayed in any psychiatric ward.

Before I ever came into nursing, in my forties, I was already
aware that I saw people in two quite distinct ways at the same
time:

I could stand back and be objective and survey a person
almost like a butterfly collector surveyed his latest specimen on
a pin: 'Ah, interesting! Look at this feature and at that . . . '

But I was conscious, too, of this being a person like myself.
One way and another I was meeting people with a whole heap
of problems. The messes that some people got into! My own life
had had just a few, and what with those and my recognition of
my own humanity - my need for love, security, independence
and mental stimulation for a start - I could warm to the people I
met.

People who work with psychiatric patients need this kind of
blend - objectivity plus warmth. I like the summary passed on
to me by my former hospital chaplain, who had himself been
taught it by a worker in a hospital: 'If you constantly become

overinvolved with your patients, you haven't the right head
for this work. If you never ever become overinvolved with a
patient, you haven't the right heart for this work.'

There have been seven subsections under this present
heading of staff-patient attitudes, each important, and all
interrelated, but isn't this idea of putting ourselves in the
patients' shoes a key to all the others? If we develop a habit so
ingrained that it becomes automatic, of asking 'How would I
feel? . . . How would I like it? . . . What would I do? . . . What
would I want?', shan't we then become much better skilled at
getting our attitudes right?

But, aha, please note: we must try to put ourselves in the
patients' shoes, not try to fit them into ours!

I learnt that years ago. I was 27. I had had an operation for
breast cancer and my wound was slow in healing. I was to have
a course of radiotherapy within a few weeks. My two children,
aged three years and ten months, were with their grandmother
in Essex, I was in our nearest big hospital in Shrewsbury, and
my husband was alone in our rented and furnished flat in
mid-Wales.

'I don't know why they keep that flat on', someone remarked
- and the remark was injudiciously passed on to me. 'They
really need just a bed-sit and a landlady now. That's what I'd
do if I were them.'

The speaker was not us, and no way were we likely to do such
a thing!

'That's what I'd do, if I were them' - mistrust that comment.
Has the speaker really asked 'What does it feel like, being *them*?
Can I put myself properly into *their* shoes?'

As people asking, 'What kind of a person has this psychiatric
illness/this psychiatric problem?', let's try to find out all we can
about our patients, in order to see them as fully in the round as
we can. To help my student nurses to do this I give each one my
'Permutations of Personality' sheet, and we talk it through. It is
a topic I find exciting every time I think about it. Every time we
talk it through there is fresh material for discussion:

'Do you know what Stella said the other day? "Do I really
have to do the washing up? Don't you realise I had nine
servants when I lived in India?" '

'Sheila's black-haired now, but that's new. She was a

peroxide blonde until she suddenly redyed it in the washroom two weeks ago.'

'Edna was telling me the other day that she studied the violin at Dartington Hall when it first opened.'

We speak about ourselves, too, in these sessions. I can speak on coming to terms with divorce and on the boost one can have as a newly married person. Last time a student recounted how, as an eight-year-old, she had overheard her future stepfather being told, 'Getting married to a widow with three kids? You must be crazy!'

'Oh, that must have hurt!', I said, knowing how I'd have felt, and bleeding for that eight-year-old.

'No! I was surprised. "What a silly person!" I thought. "We're a lovely family and he will be lucky to join us!" '

So I had to adjust my mental picture of that eight-year-old. Fatherless, about to have a stepfather, and yet marvellously secure.

A final example is one which tickled my sense of humour. Sheila is a young lady I now know outside the hospital. We had met at the Sunday Quaker meetings and had since been going to discussion evenings together. Only at the very end of those did I happen to say 'Yes, C.S. Lewis is a favourite author of mine, too. But his Narnia stories weren't written when I was young. I discovered those when my sons read them.'

'Sons? Sons? What's this about sons? I didn't even know you were married, Margaret! You don't wear a ring. Now I'll have to rebuild my picture of you all over again!'

Sheila would make a smashing psychiatric nurse. She's aware of the need to see people in the round.

This chapter has gone on and on, and is by far the longest. And because the points I have been trying to make are so important I will spell them out all over again in this summary. Not to treat the reader like a child, but in the hope that the reader will say 'Yes, that is so . . . and that . . . oh yes, how important that is. Yes, that is what I do want to put into practice and what I shall want to keep passing on to other people.'

● Patients often feel they are not getting the help they need.

● People need people. We need to relate comfortably to one another.

● Helping patients to relate to others is at the heart of caring for psychiatric patients.

● Psychiatric patients are frequently turned in on themselves. It is a major feature of their condition, closely linked to their difficulty in relating to other people.

● Everyone sees the patients as 'so selfish!' occasionally. Maybe they shouldn't, but they will scarcely be human if they never do.

● Nurses' attitudes to patients must be good before a good nurse-patient relationship can start.

● Patients are people - normal people most of the time.

● The 'golden mean' is desirable. We must recognise both the patients' normal and abnormal behaviour.

● Treating patients as normal encourages them to behave normally.

● We use a 'medical model' to describe the place where we work, the work, the workers and the residents. But 'patient' and 'ill' may be the wrong words.

● The roles of those involved in caring for psychiatric patients are complex. We need to recognise that we assume a variety of roles.

● The 'patient' role is likely to encourage dependency.

● An adult-adult approach puts the patient on a good footing.

● Very many psychiatric patients have lived with their difficulties for decades. It may therefore take time before good staff attitudes produce a good response.

● To get the balance right we need objectivity and subjectivity, detachment and warmth.

● Trying to help involves putting ourselves in the patients' shoes.

● To put ourselves in the patients' shoes we need as wide a knowledge of the patients as possible.

References

Aristotle (384-322 B.C.). *Politics*.
Berne, E. (1966). *Games People Play*, London: Deutsch.

Bible, 1 Corinthians 13: 1-3 (my paraphrase).

Donne, J. (1571-1631). *Devotions*.

Flaherty, M. (1981). 'For Mara', *The Nursing Mirror*, 26 February.

Harris, T.A. (1973). *I'm OK - You're OK*, London: Pan. (First published 1970 as *The Book of Choice*, London: Jonathan Cape.)

Jones, K. and Sidebotham, R. (1962). *Mental Hospitals at Work*, London: Routledge and Kegan Paul.

Powell, J. (1969). *Why Am I Afraid to Tell You Who I Am?*, Illinois: Argus Communications. (Also London: Fontana/Collins.)

Shakespeare, W. (1564-1616). *Merchant of Venice*, Shylock's 'I am a Jew' speech (with two words changed).

3 Patients and Staff Together

Getting to know you,
Getting to know all about you.
Getting to like you,
Getting to hope you like me.
Getting to know you,
Putting it my way
But nicely
You are precisely
My cup of tea.
Getting to know you,
Getting to feel free and easy
When I am with you,
Getting to know what to say.
Haven't you noticed
Suddenly I'm bright and breezy,
Because of all the beautiful and new
Things I'm learning about you
Day
by
day.

(From *The King and I*, Rodgers and Hammerstein, 1951)

Getting Stuck in the Office!

I am appalled by the number of statements I am making which
seem so obvious. Here's another: people who care for psychiatric patients will never get to know their patients unless they
meet them. They will not meet them properly if too much time
is spent in the ward's office.

Yet at times the office is like a magnet, even to nurses whose
preference is to be with the patients.

What happens? Alison, a nurse, has been cooking with Pauline, and talking about the appointment Pauline has the next day.

'Is the appointment at four?' asks Pauline.

'I think it's four, but I'd better check that while we think of it.'

But in the office Alison is caught up in a conversation with the sister. It begins with something the sister particularly wants to ask, goes on to something interesting enough for Alison to linger 'just a moment or two', and when the doctor arrives Alison stops on because she has information about Geoffrey to pass on to him. What is Pauline's feeling? We need to recognise this pull away from the patients, and we need to put ourselves in the patients' shoes: 'The nurses don't really like being with us. They prefer being with each other.' It is frequently not true, but it must seem so.

It frequently is true. The patients' very inability to relate easily to others makes it hard for nurses to relate easily to them. What nurse is there who never turns in sheer relief (recognised or unrecognised) to the fellow nurses who respond so easily?

There are times when the nurses have to be in the office. People like the ward sister and charge nurse often have difficulty in getting out. But student nurses, too, need to be in the office sometimes to plan their work, to say what they have been finding out amongst the patients, to talk over their findings, to learn from the experience of others, to back up their findings from the patients' notes and from textbooks, or to refute them!

But the chief place of the psychiatric nurse is with the patient. In the next pages we shall travel outwards with the patients, starting by being on the ward with the patients and gradually getting them right out for periods in the world outside the hospital.

On the Ward

WINNING THE PATIENTS' ACCEPTANCE

Notice the words used in the previous sentence - *with* the patients - that's the chief thing. But let's say it again: it is not easy to stay with patients who offer no response, complete apathy, or strongly negative responses, scowls, mutterings, 'Will you leave me alone, please!' or who get up and shoot away as the nurses join them!

How are we to handle such situations? Flexibly. There is no single rule. The patients are individuals and so must our responses be. Play the situations by ear. Be adaptable.

Allow the patient the right to be alone sometimes. Put yourselves in their shoes. This is their home for the moment, maybe for only a week or two, but it may have been their home for decades. How much privacy can they have? It will vary, but for some it is little, as I learned when I was snowed in my hospital for three nights, and spent one of them in a vacant bed to the delight and care of the dormitory's other occupants! They looked after me well, and there was perhaps a bit of teaching as well as teasing in old Ada's goodnight: 'Sleep well - and I hope you went to the toilet before you got in!'

Do not assume, however, that the patients really do not want company. Put yourselves next into the shoes of an acutely depressed patient. Perhaps her thoughts go like this:

Everything is terrible. I can't see any future for myself. I feel a complete dead-weight. These nurses will never be able to help me. And they're so busy. Calling people to see the doctors, chasing after that rather mad young man, giving out tablets and seeing to the dinners, looking after that patient who is in bed . . . there's no end to their work, poor things. I haven't even the energy or brightness to say anything when they do come. That nice young nurse - I think he said 'My name is Mike' - he's sat beside me a few times. He was glad to sit down and rest himself, I expect. If I weren't so stupid I might have talked to him. I'd have liked to have done that.

And gradually it gets through the thick hide that she has developed in her present state that Mike is seeking her out from time to time. That he actually cares about her. That he feels she is worth caring about. And then she begins to feel she may be worth caring about!

Here is another approach.

> *Sister*   I can see from your scowl that you don't like me
> Shirley. I'm sorry about that. It makes me keep away,
> and I like getting to know people and I'd like to get to
> know you a little bit really. Not if you really don't want
> me to. But your scowls do hurt me a little!

Shirley has gone on scowling at the sister for a week or
two after saying that the nurses treat the patients as if
they own them. Interestingly, she has related much
better to one of the new general student nurses. Does
she feel less taken-over by this young girl who will only
be here for eight weeks? But she now thinks about the
sister's statement and smiles in a way the sister has not
seen before.

> *Shirley*   Oh, I've felt very hurt myself. I know how it
> feels.

A week later, after a much more relaxed atmosphere
has developed between them, Shirley looks in the office
and speaks to the sister.

> *Shirley*   I'm thinking of going to the George for a
> Babycham tonight. Would you like to come?

There will be no 'miraculous cure' for Shirley immediately. But
which is nearer to the normal? Sullen scowls and lumpen
lethargy, or inviting someone to the pub?
  Play it by ear and adapt the approaches. How awful it would
be if nurses learnt to approach patients with standard patter
and the patients heard them trotting a helpful remark out
dutifully first to one patient and then another! It would not
make them feel like cared-for individuals.
  So far I've only written about approaches that might draw
the nurse and patient together. What might they actually do
when they are together?

WORKING WITH PATIENTS ON THE WARD

There are all the obviously 'work' activities. Bed-making,

washing clothes, ironing, sorting through and tidying wardrobes and drawers and a bed area, sweeping and dusting, laying tables for meals, washing-up, making tea, cooking meals and cakes.

Of course all this will vary from ward to ward and patient to patient. It may be much more important for a patient to make his bed on his own. The washing may be best done in the hospital laundry, and if done on the ward the nurse may teach a patient how to use an automatic washing machine as good preparation for popping out to a launderette. A few patients have uncomfortably immaculate bed areas; at the other extreme a few manic patients accumulate case upon case of clothes from every jumble sale they can get to. The domestic staff may feel more hampered than helped if the patients sweep or dust, or that their work is being criticised or their job at risk!

Even over a task as humdrum as bed-making, nurses learn a great deal. About the patients' ability to make a bed, for a start! And about their mental condition: their ability to concentrate, dementia perhaps, mania, depression . . . but that is not what I am thinking of primarily here. It was over bed-making when I roped Nancy in to help me make Jim's bed. It was an absolute disgrace in an otherwise reasonably homely dormitory, and not at all fair to the other occupants when they used it as a bed-sit. We were getting no help from Jim at that time, and Nancy began talking about her memories of her 'bad old days', and the tremendous aggression that used to well up inside her until it burst out in physical violence. We never saw such aggression. Why not? Partly, Nancy thought, because the nurses' attitudes provoked her a lot less. No, I did not put that idea into Nancy's head. It was Nancy's comment that made me go on considering the need for good attitudes.

GAMES ON THE WARD

As well as work on the wards there is play. In 'It beats knitting squares!' (Rhodes, 1980) the author described a range of games played on the ward. And, more importantly, why they needed to be played. For fun, whyever not! But table-tennis got a near catatonic patient making definite responses at the opposite end of the table and a smile on to her face as she rediscovered an old skill. Beggar-my-neighbour had four almost solitary patients grouped around a table. A simple crossword raised Eva's self-esteem. Try playing games with patients and see what you learn and what effect it all has on the patients. There's no end to the surprises.

Tom is a paranoid schizophrenic, if one has to pin a label on him. Sometimes it is advisable to remember that he can become sullen, suspicious and hostile to his ward staff, even though he is now highly esteemed in the job he holds out of the hospital. His chief interest is to take his hospital lady-friend to the pub where he is a first-class darts player. Unbeatable, we thought. And then Debbie, a student nurse, beat him, several times! Oh God, what a silly girl! But no, it cemented a friendship between the two, and the next time Tom was muttering angrily against the ward sister it was Debbie who was best able to distract him.

GROUP MEETINGS IN THE WARD

There are more formal ways of nurses and patients getting together. The weekly ward meeting is at present a novelty on our ward. There used to be such meetings, but they lapsed from lack of obvious interest. The patients never asked to have them. The meetings became spasmodic and then forgotten. At a doctor's insistence they have been restarted and are proving a great joy to the staff and a valuable together-time for everyone. Talking topics? Raised by the patients: the state of the loos; could they soon have another party with games like the Christmas one, as it was better than the discos; the washing-up rota (a repeated topic for discussion); how could we all stop Cindy cadging cigarettes? Raised by me, as sister: that our hospital's two wards for disturbed patients were changing their function and would no longer automatically take anyone who became very disturbed on our ward, so would everyone accept that the nurses might very occasionally have to use more sedation than normally; it would not mean that we were changing our basic way of dealing with people; we would go on trying to treat people individually. This got a marvellously supportive reaction from the patients to the staff.

At one ward meeting Stuart went on and on about 'Can't we do exercises?' So we do. Mondays to Fridays at 5 p.m. Stuart often dodges them, but since it was his idea he is the one patient we try to rope in! Some days there is scarcely space in our sun-room for all the press-ups, arm-swinging and spontaneous movement. We used a ballet-music tape one day and a lot of us became quite hilarious. 'This exercise is called "Spot the Staff!"' said our first-year student, Fiona, and Muriel, an often spiteful patient, cackled joyfully but acceptably. Some days it looks as if only the nurses will be exercising, but one or two patients will always join us.

Some ward meetings and some ward togetherness will be very clearly 'proper psychiatric hospital work', such as our Thursday afternoon group meeting for six patients, the registrar, and as many nurses as can come; the behaviour-therapy project that Jacqui, a nurse, and Greg, a patient, have worked out and that Julie and Linda, nurses, have jointly worked out with Michael, a patient. When the tutors, student nurses, ward staff, patients, psychologists and doctors have combined in such projects to see if better help can be given to patients it has been great! It so raises my morale as a sister. Too often we seem to do too little.

PATIENTS WITH PATIENTS

Whilst planning regimes of therapeutic treatment, we must recognise that any nurse-patient togetherness can be 'therapeutic'. And also nurse-patient-patient togetherness. Because out of that comes the following:

Scene A ward's sitting room. Four patients are sitting around the table, playing dominoes. The sister and a nurse pass the open door. They gasp.

Sister It's unbelievable!
Nurse Which of them organised that, do you think?

That domino group afterwards regularly filled in odd patches of time with a game. Teresa, a Polish refugee with a horrid life history, was the organiser.

Those four patients had all been in hospital or abnormal living conditions for 40 years or more. They had become very used to waiting for instructions as to what to do.

At first it was the nurses who had gathered up the domino players. Six or seven enjoyed dominoes. Or did when they had been shown how to play it. Some remembered it from childhood, some grasped it quickly, some showed an odd response to 'Put that six next to the other six' - you would think that instruction was simple enough when it was also being repeatedly demonstrated, but Helen persisted in lining up the dominoes alongside one another instead of end to end.

Against their background of a lack of initiative, a disinclination to form groups, and a difficulty in playing even a simple game, Teresa's formation of the domino team was indeed marvellous.

But there is a further point to be made now. We very readily see the patients as loners. The days have not yet gone of chairs lined up against walls and patients sitting in isolation, side by side. Indeed this is often still the hospital norm. Another reason for the nurses to get out of the office and among the patients is so that they may become aware of the relationships that do exist between patient and patient. The same point has to be made here as was made about seeing the patients' normality: we have to look for this or we shall fail to see it. There are already patient-patient relationships which we can help to grow. If Maggy and Irene are quietly buddies, in their own odd way, when Maggy is drawn into a game, or to make a cake, include Irene in too. Instead of sitting and talking just to Irene, or watching the television with Irene, get the chairs dragged round so that you are a threesome: yourself, Irene and Maggy. Or become a fivesome for chatting together, once you've realised that Teresa, Maggy, Irene and Geraldine play dominoes together.

The nurse may often have to initiate the building of relationships through nurse-patient togetherness. But a patient-patient friendship is better for all sorts of reasons.

Around the Hospital

FREEDOM TO ROAM

Patients are not confined to their wards! That is an obvious statement to the nurses who read this book. But it is still far from obvious to those who know nothing or little about psychiatric hospitals. One instance out of many I've heard at first hand:

> A *new assistant in the patients' central restaurant* I can't help laughing when I go along the hospital corridors these days. Do you know, the day I came for my interview for this job I had no idea that the people I was meeting along the corridors were patients. I assumed that they would all be shut away on their wards!

Let's clear the exceptions out of the way first. The patients who have been most recently admitted may be asked to stay on their own wards at first. For the outsider it even has to be spelled out sometimes that a ward equals a home, with all the rooms of a home and more, and that a ward does *not* equal a dormitory with patients in bed! Very rarely, it may be best for a longer-stay temporarily disturbed patient to stay on his/her ward. It is true that the most handicapped psychogeriatrics may seldom leave their wards, though this may well be a tragedy and a failure of management, and not an inevitability.

But, with these exceptions, the patients are free to move around the whole hospital area, and this is likely to be large: many buildings spread around acres of land. The two hospitals I know have a tea-room, a church, cricket and football fields, staff social club, nurses' homes (large hostels as well as small family houses), great stretches of 'park' and wonderful long-established trees, and roads, buses and car parks!

To pick up a point made in the last section, it is often good for the patients to get out of the ward on their own, or with friends that they have on other wards, to get away from their nurses and their fellow-patients. In quite normal situations out of the hospital two people who are too much together can rub one another up the wrong way. How much more can this happen between 30 patients in a psychiatric ward! But do nurses recognise that well enough yet? How would we like to be one of the patients on a ward day after day, night after night? So be it, if they choose to wander at will around the whole hospital village - or however they see it. And if nurses wish to modify their freedom to roam a little, let's be sure it is to put something better in its place.

Why might those of us who care for psychiatric patients want to get them off the ward to activities of our suggesting? There are several answers and I may not have them all.

EXPANDING HORIZONS

In 'Looking for normality on a psychogeriatric ward' (Putnam, 1974) I described how dementing 'Mrs M' was entranced by the hustle-bustle of life in the hospital's main corridor on a day she had 'escaped' from her usually locked ward. (Locked for her own safety as a wanderer.) She could have found her own way back, or have been returned by someone who found her wandering, and her ward's nurses would have had no idea of the pleasure her escapade had given her. She might have been fetched back by a nurse without eyes or ears and who would have failed to see her pleasure, even though she was radiant. We have to develop a habit of looking and listening in order to see and to hear.

GIVING PATIENTS MORE NORMAL EXPERIENCES

We must help them maintain or relearn how to handle such experiences. For example, it was once common practice for the patients' money to be spent for them, a bulk order - fancy cakes, tinned fruit and cream, chocolate, sweets, talc, nice soaps and shampoos - being sent from the hospital shop without the patients being involved at all. Obviously this could lead to a misuse of the patients' money. But more positively, how much better it is for the patients themselves to do the shopping. Preferably at 'real' shops in the 'real' world! Failing that, at a hospital shop that is as much like an outside shop as possible.

What a growth there has been in giving the patients normal

experience within the hospital! The hairdressing salons, banks that look like banks, a tea-room purpose-built outside the main building. The development of social therapy departments that help to provide activities for the hours when they are most needed, that is, for the evenings and the weekends.

In my present hospital the term 'social skills' is used a great deal, and I would like to debate this term a little. There is a danger, I believe, in the use of technical terms. A technical term is, at its best, a form of shorthand. 'Social skills' puts in two words a very great deal: an easy, natural handling of a range of situations, an ability to relate well to the other people in those situations with the ability to look at the other people and to speak up clearly and intelligibly, an ability to cope with the unexpected without panic . . . and there is more.

The dangers in the use of such terms? That something which should have become instinctive becomes too self-conscious. What man-in-the-street says 'My social skills are excellent'? In fact, a large number of men-in-the-street have poor social skills and yet get by in the everyday world. There are those who care for psychiatric patients whose social skills are poorer than those of the patients themselves. Is it an impertinence to assume that we should or could teach social skills to all the patients?

A second danger: an assumption that if one knows the term and uses the term repeatedly one is thereby magically doing the work? That is cynical. I accept that it is good to be aware of the need for social skills, but I would like to hear a little less of them and see nurses getting out and about the hospital alongside their patients, setting an example of normal behaviour and quietly helping the patients to behave normally.

Philip was a tall, bright-eyed, intelligent 40 year old who mingled easily in the crowds in the town where he frequently took himself. He didn't say very much on the ward. But he once opened up and told a nurse 'Do you know, there was one nurse who tried to run a course for us on How To Get On With Others. The first lesson was "How To Say Yes And No Nicely!" '

Another time the dentist was to show a film on the ward. It was in connection with Self-help Groups. On that occasion Philip said 'A film about how to clean our teeth? Good God! I know how to clean my teeth! I just don't do it; that's all!'

MORE WORK EXPERIENCE?

There is much disagreement between nurses and patients, and between nurses and nurses, about the 'work' to which the patients are directed. There can easily be serious ward versus occupational or industrial therapy department strife, if this is not seen as bad and stopped!

Two main reasons are given for directing the patients to such work: it helps to prepare them for a job outside the hospital; and by making them concentrate on their work it prevents them from drifting off into their dream worlds or listening to their voices, or however we see that.

Again and again I hear student nurses speak up: 'It's rubbish really! The work areas are so unlike those of the real world.' 'Look at the amounts they earn there - two or three pounds a week, perhaps five or so if they work extremely well. And it doesn't stop them drifting off. The good workers learn to do their job automatically and go on thinking their private thoughts. The poor workers keep stopping their work or they make a mess of their work so that it has to be redone by someone else.'

On this whole topic I put myself into a series of 'other shoes': those of the patients, the occupational and industrial therapy staff, the people for whom the work is done, the nurses, the non-nursing administrators and the patients' relatives:

The patients frequently complain that the work offered is repetitive and boring. On the whole it is.

The OT and IT staff complain that the patients lack concentration and motivation. They do. The staff tell us that they have great difficulty in obtaining even the work that they have. That's often true.

The businessmen would say that they are under no obligation to occupy the patients in psychiatric hospitals. Their job is to run a profitable business. Their interest is to get the work done quickly and accurately.

The nurses - especially the ward's permanent staff - feel they are failing if the patients sit around all day on the ward. Greg actually says 'What shall I do? Tell me what to do. It's so boring. It's awful.' Greg has been bored for about 35 years out of his 48. He is an exception both in his voicing of his feelings on this subject and in the degree to which he can resist every effort to occupy him!

Administrators and the relatives cannot imagine the problems of this 'work' situation. 'You say the patient lacks money. But he could earn some!' 'You say that Joan will not attend industrial therapy. But she could be made to go!' It sounds simple enough, and I would think like this were I not a psychiatric nurse.

As part of a nursing management course I took as a project 'Socialising the Solitary'. One of the people to whom I showed it wrote:

> I think stimulus and occupation very valuable even if the patients would rather get on without them. But I wonder if they can ever be a substitute for work - the sort of work that gives the worker not money but a sense of his/her own value in the society. The sense of the good estimation of others could result in an altered estimate by themselves. The work the patients do is absolutely not designed to make them aware of their place in the world, as of value. Providing such work is probably an impossibility! But anything else is second-best, I think!

Some patients are fortunate enough to find work which is meaningful for them. From my present ward Muriel goes out from 1 to 4 p.m. to clear tables and wash up in the large tea-room, and Steve is a bed-maker on a psychogeriatric ward. 'Well, it is useful, isn't it!' he says, before anyone can say that this is not a man's work. Two patients have satisfying jobs outside the hospital and some do feel that their regular occupational and industrial therapy is worth while. Edna has been stuck lately on knitting scarves in spider stitch for all her favourite people. There is nothing wildly exciting about her 'work', except that it is her own choice of occupation and she greatly enjoys it, and 18 months ago she was curled up too often in a foetal position or hiding in a corner of the loo.

To make the overall point of this whole chapter again, which may have got a little sunk beneath all the tempest-tossing that 'work' can cause: unless the nurses are with the patients enough in all the areas to which they go off the ward, they cannot properly know them. Just as a game on the ward with a patient reveals the unexpected, so does any off-the-ward activity.

There are many examples of this lesson in the literature, including one which involved a student nurse on her very first ward discovering how differently an apparently dementing and psychotic patient chose to behave in an area where she was happier (Lloyd, 1981).

So, mental illness involves the breakdown of relationships, and our task is to help our patients to relate more comfortably to other people. To do that we need to know our patients in the round, as whole people, and that involves knowing them off the ward as well as on it.

A QUESTION OF CHOICE

What is to be done about patients who choose not to be involved in our attempts to help them? Of course one feels sad about the few patients who strenuously resist all attempts to get them to join in events off the ward. And yet, out of the 30 patients on the ward where I was first a sister, one of the few who is now happily out of hospital was a Jewish woman we always left behind, no matter where we were going. And, when we were presented with a load of her belongings, including a stack of family photographs that she did not want to see, and put those alongside her reluctant statement 'No family now. Had family once. All dead.', her wish to cling to her favourite seat in her ward home was understandable.

Out of the Hospital

UNFAMILIAR SITUATIONS

I had thought my chief point in this book was to underline the need of psychiatric patients, and indeed everyone for developing good, meaningful relationships. This expands to: patients have difficulty in making good relationships, and our main job as psychiatric nurses is to help them. But a new point has sidled in from time to time: that patients often need help in handling experiences, especially ones which are familiar to ordinary people but not familiar to them.

Take crossing the street! Rita dreaded being out in the nearest town. She said so. Rita did go out occasionally, but it was only out in the street with Rita that the nurses fully appreciated her terror of the traffic. And she was only 38. But just imagine how much emptier the roads were 20 years earlier when she was 18 and she first came into the hospital.

Or can nurses imagine that? Even those of us who are older forget how different it all used to be, since we often go out into the gradually changing world. My husband took two sets of photographs all around the Welsh market town where we lived for 13 years, as an exercise with his schoolboys. The greatest impact the photos made was in the difference in the traffic; that astonished us. There had always been plenty of traffic, we would have said, but in the first set of photos the streets looked nearly empty.

I must resist the temptation in this book to give long lists of ways in which the nurses can get the patients out of hospital for the day. What I must say is: be keenly alert to all the difficulties the patient has in a wide variety of situations, and help them to overcome them.

Some of our experiences with the patients will be so embarrassing that we can't fail to miss them. There was I sauntering down the High Street with three patients, trying to look like four people who shopped together every day, even though Edie was moaning noisily about her feet. Then Elsie's knickers fell down. I was so busy listening to Edie that I only realised what was happening to Elsie when she pulled her knickers up in full view of everyone. Oh the embarrassment! What was worse, they fell down again, and she would have repeated the full saga all over again!

'Step out of them, Elsie, fold them up, and put them - where?' A lot more fuss from Elsie till I found a plastic carrier bag. But we now had Elsie's proclamations of 'When can I put my knickers on?' added to Edie's 'My feet are killing me.' Only when we had found a loo and a safety pin were we able to get back to the task of looking like a group of normal shoppers.

On another occasion, three of us were choosing some ornaments for the ward. Only then did I become fully aware of Marion's awkward gait and the likelihood that she might lurch into the islands of china in a crowded display. Marion seemed oblivious of the danger. She was not used to finding china in front of her, to the back of her, and to the side of her. She was used to large and rather bare hospital rooms.

I said that helping the patients to handle experiences properly was an additional task. But of course it is part of the complex skill of relating well to other people. In the hospital no-one would have been outraged if Elsie pulled her knickers up. It would just have been Elsie being spontaneous. 'Oh, Elsie!' we might have laughed, reprovingly. But people who did not know Elsie and who were unused to such an action would immediately feel anxious and hostile. 'What else might such a strange lady do? Take her away! Protect us!' Put yourselves in the shoes of the outsiders. Marion in the china department was steered away gently and nothing was broken. But if it was, how would you have reacted as the salesman?

For everyone's sake, to make life more equable, to make it possible for people to relate well to people, the patients need help in handling normal experiences. And they can only properly be helped by having the experiences to handle.

Grab every opportunity, like, for example, a ward party. It must be the patients who help to write the shopping list and who shop. Yes, it is so much quicker for the staff to get the goods. Yes, we are frequently short-staffed and who will look after the 27 back at the hospital if one or two nurses are out with two or three patients?

Our thinking is often muddled, isn't it? Isn't there a sneaky feeling that the nurse is having a treat if she's able to go out with one patient? Fancy! Denise, the nurse, sat in a hairdressers for a couple of hours while Janette had the Afro she had been coveting. Even I, as ward sister, first thought 'What a waste of Denise's time!' and said 'You could take a textbook.' How terrible! Fortunately Denise was a better psychiatric nurse than I was at that moment. I saw from her grin that it would not do. Afterwards she told me how she and Janette had, without prior planning, managed to look like friends. Janette, a very difficult young lady indeed at times, handled the situation well, and she

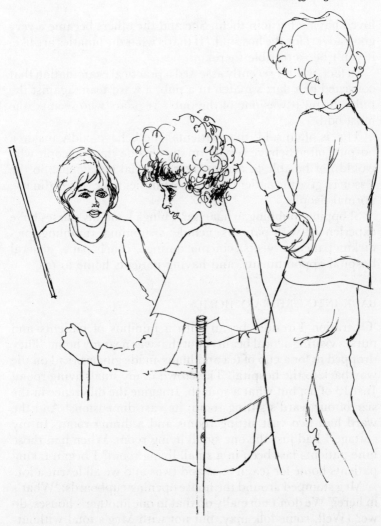

was extremely grateful to Denise for not making it clear that
'This is a patient from the mental hospital.'

And yet, occasionally it is good for the outsider to know that
this is a psychiatric patient. Many people are very helpful. One
ward of mostly elderly women had a favourite pub in the
country and every two or three weeks the hospital's minibus
would take eight or nine patients and two or three nurses there.
Fat Lily, aged 80, loved those outings and the pub's regulars

loved having her join them. She and the others became a very good advert for the hospital. 'If that's what the lunatics are like, it can't be so terrible there!'

In fact, when I recently assessed a practical examination that consisted of a dart's match in a pub, a ward team against the pub's team, it was one of the pub's regulars who seemed the most odd.

This is often said: that patients who behave oddly inside a hospital often behave very normally outside among people who would not be able to accept their unsocial behaviour. So the lesson is: give the patients the opportunities to be very ordinary, normal people.

Shopping, pubbing, what else? Things I and my nurses have experienced with patients include: swimming, rambling, picnicking, theatre visits, cinema outings, coach trips, general hospital appointments, and having patients home to tea.

BACK INTO ORDINARY HOMES

'Operation Fireside' began with a minibus of patients and nurses visiting a local beauty spot that was near my home. They dropped in for a cup of tea and home-made gingerbread on the way back to the hospital. The crowd in my small living room! Just 13 of us, but what a squash. Imagine the difference in the size of our ward's sitting room: its vast dimensions! And the ward had two vast sitting rooms and a dining room. In my cottage I had just the one small living room. When had those nine patients last been in a small living room? I began taking patients home for tea in ones and twos and we all learnt a lot.

Meg stomped around the house opening cupboards: 'What's in here?' We don't normally do that in one another's houses, do we? (Well, some folk may, but not with Meg's total without-your-leave approach.) But how do we treat the patients' wardrobes and lockers? Meg was, when I thought about it, treating me as I had treated her. Fortunately, as there had never been any malice in my 'What have you got in here, Meg?', Meg looked in my wardrobes with the same childlike curiosity. But it is not 'normal' behaviour.

Some patients, who in a hospital setting looked less normal, in the home setting became more normal. Lame Eva, who so often jerked about, disturbed by her threatening voices, sat in utter peace for a whole hour and a half with the cat on her lap. 'What lovely things you have!' she said. 'Things? What things?' I wondered. And I looked at my possessions with a new eye and contrasted the patients' normal surroundings. That purchase of china with Marion came after I told the League of Friends about Eva's comment and they gave us £50 for 'things'.

OUT WITH RELATIVES

Another normal event. Our hospital's wards were area-organised. Our ward's relatives nearly all came from 20 miles to the east of the hospital. It was an inspired charge nurse who said 'Instead of getting the relatives to come to us, why can't we go to them?' So we hired a big coach and made a park a Sunday afternoon meeting place. Imagine our arrival:

'There's Mavis and Ron! Hullo, hullo!' called old Aggie as she spotted her niece and nephew-in-law.

'I can see Ted!' said Joyce as her brother moved forward.

'Where's my brother?' asked Theresa. And there he was.

So many little groups: daughter with parents: sisters with sisters and brother-in-law; mothers with daughters, sons-in-law and grandchildren; aunts with nieces; sisters with brothers. The whole party dispersed in small groups until it was time to meet for the party tea in the restaurant's private room.

Patients with nurses and all those who care for them. That's what this chapter is about. And patients with outsiders, known and unknown. Patients learning to handle the experiences that for others are so familiar that they need little thought.

THE PATIENT ALONE

Finally, I want to pick up a point made in both the earlier 'On the ward' and 'Around the hospital' sections - at times it will be best to let the patient go it alone, or with fellow-patients: shopping, to the pub, to visit a friend or relative. My best experience of that to date was when Pauline, who at times has been notorious within my present hospital, had to see the Ear, Nose and Throat specialist at the general hospital. She was not going to be taken, she told us. She would go alone or not at

all. Help! What were we to do? We have had complaints from
that hospital when the accompanying nurse has not known the
patient in depth. What if there was no accompanying nurse?
But Pauline can speak well for herself. I rang the consultant and
told him so. I said that while she could be difficult with us she
would very much want to show herself at her best with the
general nurses and doctors and the other patients. That it
would be of immense benefit to her if he could treat her as an
ordinary person. That she was quite intelligent and would
appreciate any explanations he chose to give her. The consultant thanked me for ringing and sounded grateful that he was
treated as if he could handle a psychiatric patient well. Pauline
returned from all her visits to him, before and after an
operation, full of the good way in which she had been treated.
She was kept fully informed about all that was wrong and how it
would be put right and what the post-operative effect might be.
And the consultant communicated with the ward by post, just
as he would have done with an outside patient and her GP.

This is what we are aiming at: first-class relationships with
others.

Away for the Night

IN RELATIVES' HOMES

The biggest jump the psychiatric patients, particularly those
who have spent some time in hospital, have to make is from
being with staff and fellow-patients who know them and who
accept them as they are, including all their odd ways, to being
among strangers who cannot. So it is the previous step, getting
out of the hospital for shopping trips or for day trips, that is
likely to be the biggest hurdle. After that, staying out for a few
days will extend their experiences and the variety of situations
with which they have to cope, but the worst hurdle, of being
among strangers, is over.

Some patients, while still clearly very odd at times, will have
had frequent nights away from the hospital. This is often
because they can go from the shelter and security of the hospital

to the shelter and security of the home of an understanding and tolerant relative.

I earlier quoted Nancy's wish to have regular nights out at her sister's home. She spelled out for herself her need to belong. Nancy had a strong sense of 'family' even though she had been so long away. Her sister came twice a week to visit her, her brother came on Sunday afternoons. Nancy already visited her sister a little, dropping in for a coffee after shopping and occasionally going for the day on Saturday. But she regularly got that wrong. To Nancy's mind the day began at 7 a.m. No, this was not because we regularly hauled her out of bed every day at 7 a.m. On Saturdays and Sundays she could lie in all morning if she wished, and she was one of those who often got up later then. But she was determined to make the most of her whole day at her sister's, and she would be nicely dressed and ready to walk there after an early breakfast. It was no good our saying that if someone was coming to our homes 'for the day' we'd not really expect them before half-past ten or eleven. 'My sister does. She will expect me at half-past eight.'

And, of course, by now June did expect Nancy at half-past eight. That had become a pattern. Getting a different pattern established, to include a night away, a visit from Saturday coffee-time until Sunday evening, might have been a useful way of breaking the less normal pattern.

And why might it be good to break the less normal pattern? It should be possible to have flexibility in life. But in this case the very early arrival was not the choice of both June and Nancy but settled by Nancy's dogged determination. And, at the time of writing, Nancy's dogged determination is preventing June accepting her for a night away. Nancy has quietly but firmly said from time to time that she sees herself living with her sister one day, especially now that June is widowed. Stepping into Nancy's shoes it does seem perfectly reasonable: her sister lives alone in a whole house, and Nancy herself lives in a huge institution, her physically violent outbursts long past, and the staff all praise her for being 'so very much better these days' and echo her hope that 'before long it might be possible to live outside'. But I can also step into June's shoes and not wish to have a still somewhat awkward sister suddenly living with me.

It must hurt Nancy that several of her fellow-patients on my ward go home so regularly. Indeed, Ian has come to spend much more time at home than he does in the hospital, even though it is clear to Nancy, as to all of us, that he is still very bizarre at times. Ian is in his twenties and still has his parents. But Shirley and Keith are in their forties, as Nancy is, and they too have a parent they go home to. And Elizabeth who is about the same age does go home to a sister!

AWAY WITH STAFF

Alternative means must be found to get some patients away from the hospital for a night or two. The same is true of the staff themselves. However much those who work in psychiatric hospitals enjoy their work (and I do), how good it is to leave the hospital at the end of a shift! Imagine never ever sleeping away, and always going to bed in a dormitory, and quite probably still in a dormitory without bed-curtains!

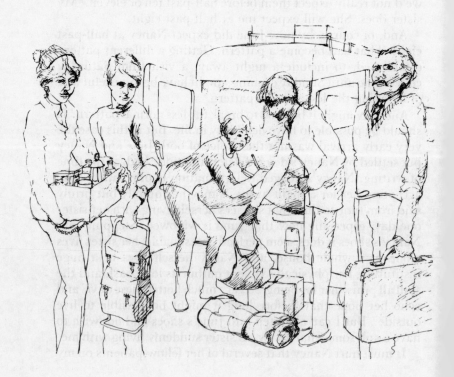

Twice last year Nancy went camping. The roof-rack and some of the seats of the hospital's invaluable minibus were piled high with tents and suitcases, food and Calor gas cookers. I pay high tribute to those who organise such trips. Perhaps the more they happen the easier they become, but I know they never 'just happen'. They take time and energy and persistence and money. And they usually require a qualified nurse in the group. But a qualified nurse who actually knows that group of patients and who can be spared from the wards and who is prepared to leave his or her own family for the weekend may be hard to find.

Holidays away are becoming more a feature of psychiatric hospitals. In the distant past, a period before my start in the 1970s, there were hospital exchanges, patients and staff swapping wards from hospital to hospital, seeing new faces and new areas. But it is the 'normal' we are now in search of. And from time to time reports of patients' holidays appear in, for example, the nursing press: a week under canvas, self-catering holidays, pony-trekking, holidays abroad. All emphasise the value it has been to the patients to get right away from the institution.

Here are a few extracts from my report about one such holiday written for the information of the hospital's non-participating staff:

Who was to go? It was obvious from the very first that we couldn't have coped with 30 patients plus even a modest number of supporting staff, even if they had all been persuadable (and they most definitely would not have been persuadable, and it would not have been our ward policy to press-gang them into coming). We ended with 10 - and this I think was ideal.

At first we thought our younger folk, recently in hospital, must go. They must be reminded how good life can be outside. In the end we took entirely patients who had been in the hospital for years. With only one exception they had all been in a hospital (and this hospital for the most part) for 30 or 40 years. Time flies - even Maureen who is still only in her mid-fifties has just managed to clock up her thirty years. And Lily too, even though she did not need a hospital at all till she was nearly fifty!

Programme of events. Obviously this was best looked at in advance and preferably on the spot. I made several trips and drafted an outline programme. It was intended as a rough guide. Flexibility is one of my ward-management principles, but in fact we stuck pretty closely to the programme, and why not? A lot of thought had gone into it to get the balance right. But this please note: we functioned for the most part in small groups. The only times we all went anywhere together were on the two bus outings. Drifting around in small groups was marvellous: myself with Amy and Lily to Lily's daughter's home; Marlene and Mary and I to the Owl Pottery because we had discovered that Mary particularly likes owls - and as we passed St Mary's Church the organist was practising so we slipped in and listened a while; Audrey, Sarah, Marlene and Gill with just Edith and Maria to listen to the band on Wednesday evening before dropping in for a drink on the way home - it had been great, they said, and people had been dancing on the grass around the bandstand; Sarah and Michael in the pool with Maureen (her first swim for 30 years) with everyone cheering as Sarah took her arms right away and held them up while Maureen completed the width on her own. And so on. Small things mainly - but things totally out of the patients' everyday life.

So many tales. I could go on and on with stories galore. I could describe the Centre in detail (the old Grammar School, now carpeted, brightly painted and curtained, with duvets and an understanding that some of its mainly young visitors may be incontinent!). I could describe some of the other guests: French children, handicapped Anglo-Austrians (some English, some Austrians), Boys Brigade boys, 21 children between 6 and 11 years from a Catholic school in Peckham - we all got on fabulously.

I will tell you our three anxious moments. And there were only three in the whole week.

(1) The embarrassment on the first evening when we were building sandpies on the beach and one of our group stepped to one side, drew up her skirt and pulled down her knickers and weed. We made sure that only happened the once! The town is well-equipped with

loos, so that was OK. (But our hospital grounds are not, and this is where they have learnt that habit.)

(2) The manager of the cinema insisted on seeing all our Old Age Pensioners before he'd admit them at half-price. We had done our best to get the tickets in advance, but he was adamant. Result: the last to arrive went in in the dark. The manager said 'Give me your hand, madam.' But that madam hates being touched so she pushed him away and told him what she thought of him. Fortunately it was only the supporting film and rather dull at that and the audience seemed to enjoy the diversion. Afterwards Sarah apologised to him - and he gracefully responded by apologising to her for not helping over the tickets.

(3) On the last night one of our patients went into a series of fits at 2 a.m. By 2.45 a.m. the doctor had been, sat quietly beside her for a moment or two while we assessed the situation - it wasn't wholly certain at first that they were fits. Then she had one clear fit. He gave a valium i.v. injection, and very shortly indeed she was round. I hope no-one will say that she shouldn't have gone.

A rather sad PS. It was a little like Christmas on the last evening. Little presents were being exchanged all round. The volunteers' group gave a small gift to everyone, and we had a small thank-you present for them too. Mary and Maureen were crying a little as they went to bed, and Lizzie and Amy were both volunteering that they didn't want to go back to the hospital.

I felt shaken by that. I have always maintained that the hospital is like a happy village. Now it really hit me that they had a real taste of being teated as ordinary people for a whole week. Was it that they did not want to go back to being second-class citizens?

When they got back I thought I'd been wrong. They were glad to see their long-time companions. Edith had brought several gifts for the ones left behind (and no mementoes for herself.) Others showed their own acquisitions. They were welcomed by the others who had missed them. But the next day Edith broke down and cried and said 'It's been such a wonderful week. It was marvellous spending so much time at my sister's house. You've no idea what it's like being in here. I feel so shut away. Do you think I'll have to stay here all the rest of my life?'

Sequel to that holiday: Edith inside the hospital was often an exceedingly strange person, one of the ward's most exasperating, as she was not obviously psychotic. In her mid-fifties she would almost literally dance round the staff, grimacing and repeating 'I am all right, nurse, aren't I?' She needed an incredible amount of help, dashing at everything she did; when dressing the clothes often went on in random order and back to front or inside out. She had already begun to improve after a review of her medication and with persistent encouragement and less showing of our very natural exasperation. After the week's holiday we pressed for her to be tried in outside accommodation. Merely to be thought capable of it further raised her morale, and at the time of writing she has been out for a year.

References

Lloyd, R. (1981). 'Wanted - A change of attitude'. *The Nursing Mirror*, 9 September.

Putnam, M. (1974). 'Looking for normality on a psychogeriatric ward', *The Nursing Mirror*, 19 September.

Rhodes, M. (1980). 'It beats knitting squares!' *The Nursing Mirror*, 31 January.

Rodgers, R. and Hammerstein, O. (1951). *The King and I*, New York: Williamson Music Inc.

4 Patients and Diagnoses

The Desire for a Diagnosis

DO STAFF WANT TO 'PARTICULARISE'?

Is there a very orderly streak in man which drives us to particularise? I was watching 'University Challenge' the other evening. 'What's this?' asked Bamber Gascoigne as a picture came up on the screen. 'And this?' A deer and a deer, I thought. But no, one was a Thompson's gazelle and one was something else. It reminded me of a wonderful character who paused to admire a flower in our garden. 'What's that?' 'A dahlia', I said, proud that I knew, because I wasn't much of a gardener then. 'I know it's a dahlia!' he said. 'What variety?'

I am not against this liking for detail. The buddleias in our garden were alive with butterflies and I was glad to distinguish red admirals, peacocks and tortoiseshells.

The greater our interest, the greater our desire for detail. Kraepelin saw not just people whose minds appeared to be failing, but some whose minds appeared to be failing particularly early, calling this 'Dementia praecox'. Bleuler looked at it differently and gave it a new name: 'the schizophrenias'. Plural, because he saw it as much more complex, containing variations. (The reader is referred to Mayer-Gross et al. (1954) for references to Kraepelin and Bleuler.) In 1973 in my first year of training we were still sweating over the details of the four main classes of schizophrenia: simple, hebephrenic, catatonic and paranoid, not to mention paraphrenia and the schizoid personalities. It even turned out from her ancient notes that dear old simple Annie had 'oligophrenia'. (Did that mean that she was, like Winnie-the-Pooh, 'of little brain' and equally as loveable?) I have - very recently too - been shown a modern list of mental illnesses that breaks this group down still further.

The same goes for psychopaths. I have 1974 notes about: the constitutional, the reactive, the trained and the untrained. To be honest, I doubt if those were ever 'proper names' for them; they were probably the 'nicknames' as it were, given by our lecturer, quite helpfully too. In 1980 as I tried better to understand certain of our patients who were 'young, not obviously ill, but determined to remain in hospital' (see Chapter 6, under 'Fifty niggles . . . ') I was making notes from Silvano Arieti's (1978) conclusions: that psychopaths might be pseudopsychopaths, idiopathic (subdivided into 'simple' and 'complex'), dyssocial and paranoiac.

Often nurses argue over the classification of their patients, debating diagnoses among themselves and disagreeing with the doctors either to their faces or behind their backs. 'Schizophrenic, my foot! He's a psychopath!' 'Hysterical reaction? But it's obvious she's schizophrenic.' I doubt if nurses will ever completely stop doing this. Knowing, and getting something right, is so deeply satisfactory!

A label satisfies the statisticians too. The Medical Records Department want to know why Belinda Jones has been admitted. We could tell them she is a 'Relapsed schizophrenic'. I am pleased that they are beginning to accept 'Social admission' for their charts instead, and seem to understand my further explanation that this former patient with a residue of slight strangeness could manage very nicely out of hospital if she and her aging mother were not cooped up alone so much in a small house. 'She won't be here very long. It will just give each of them a break for a while. And she will be going home every Friday afternoon till Monday morning.'

PATIENTS WANT ACCEPTABILITY

One consultant who had worked in a university town claimed there was a flurry of would-be schizophrenics as examinations approached. That may seem astonishing until one adds that those undergraduates would see 'schizophrenia' as a real illness and acceptable. Something for which they could not be held accountable, like failing to study.

I told earlier how Peter nearly strangled a nurse. If a diagnosis has to be fixed, Peter is probably a schizophrenic. Owing to a combination of mistakes by several people he saw a piece of paper on which was written 'Peter - lazy and slovenly' just at a time when he was failing to receive the phenothiazines which had formerly kept him stable. In Peter's case we nurses were shattered by our folly. We were lucky that both the nurse who was attacked and Peter himself came through this without lasting ill-effect. Possibly Peter would prefer to see himself as 'schizophrenic', if it were very well explained to him. He certainly objected to 'lazy and slovenly'. 'How dare you let your nurses write such things about me!' he said, shoving the paper towards me and thumping it.

Cindy, however, objected to 'schizophrenic'. She clearly interpreted it as 'severely and lunatically strange'. She was pouring herself tea in her usual disorganised way. 'Cindy,' I said, 'do try to keep your mind on what you're doing. Stop being so - schizophrenic', I settled for. Wrongly, perhaps. It was a spur-of-the-moment choice, and a degree experimental. What would she say? She was furious and shouted and buzzed around the ward like a distraught bluebottle for half an hour or so.

'I'm sorry, Cindy. I shouldn't have said that. I don't even see you as a schizophrenic. I see you as Cindy.'

Nevertheless I believe some patients do like their labels. The manic-depressive particularly? They may not like having to live with their mood-swings, but in the absence of a cure it may be easier to say 'I can't help it. I'm a manic-depressive' and feel that something chemical is out of balance and that it is a recognised illness, rather than to feel one should fight the elation or the gloom every time, or, even more frighteningly, to feel one is 'going out of one's mind'.

RELATIVES WANT REASSURANCE

I shall be trying to step into the relatives' shoes in Chapter 7. Here I ask a few questions. Don't a lot of relatives, parents especially, worry in case they have been somehow to blame for their son's or daughter's strangeness? And don't husbands and wives worry similarly about their mentally unhappy partners? Have any of us been quite guilt-free since Freud? Before Freud we could blame people's oddities onto God, or the Devil. Freud opened our eyes as to what people can do to people.

The relatives are in a particularly difficult cleft where

diagnoses are concerned. Which do they most want to hear? That the patients are basically all right and that nothing is physically wrong, but that they behave as they do because their lives have upset them? Or do the relatives want to hear that it is a genetic illness? That John is like this because, if they look into it, they will realise he had a grandfather and an aunt who were also strange, and that it is in the family - and possibly in John's children, if he now has some? The relatives will certainly be asking 'What exactly is the matter?'

The Case Against Diagnosing

THE DANGER OF THE LABEL

I have written already (in Chapter 3, under 'Around the hospital') that there is a danger of believing that if one knows a term and uses the term repeatedly one is thereby magically doing the work. Similarly I feel that there is a danger of believing that, if one has clearly identified the illness, one has thereby magically effected a cure. Or been absolved from trying.

No, maybe no-one is consciously that silly. And yet sometimes we talk as if *the* task is to get the label right.

Edith had a very odd gait and great jerkiness. I had worked on the wards with two patients with Huntington's Chorea previously, so I could see why my fellow student, Susan, thought that Edith might have it. But I knew it had already been discussed with the doctors several times in her many years in hospital.

The sister was fuming one day. Susan had written a query about Huntington's into Edith's nursing notes.

'We must get this Huntington's business settled once and for all,' said the sister.

But that was not possible. And of little practical help if we had, either to Edith or to her family. Her daughter had already had two children. Of course, it might have improved people's attitudes to Edith. It might have made them more understanding and considerate. But, then, I had heard nurses being impatient and judgemental even with the two diagnosed Huntington's: 'She doesn't have to do that. She can help herself more. She is very demanding.'

In some cases the 'right label' may horribly prejudice the nurse - and society. 'He is a psychopath' can be a terrible label to wear. Nothing good that that person does will ever be seen as genuine and any hint of awkwardness will provoke a 'There you are. He's at it again. Typical. Watch him. He's dangerous.'

Take Martine. She had been in Broadmoor for 10 years before being allowed, with many restrictions, to a hospital nearer her home. True, she was manipulative! She could charm the students into seeing her as very interesting and turn them against the permanent staff when they said 'There you are. She's at it again. Typical.' True, she was dangerous at times. Doreen's broken leg was undoubtedly caused by Martine's pushing her down a flight of stairs.

And yet?

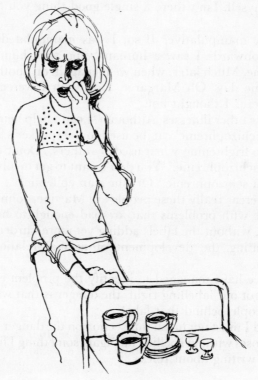

At one stage I too found Martine repulsive. I knew I was not supposed to be judgemental, but I loathed her foul stories. One day a conversation that included us both developed like this:

Martine   You don't really like me, Margaret, do you?
Me   No, not really.
Martine   Why not?
Me   I can't stand those horrible stories you so enjoy telling to upset the others. Yuch.
Martine   And what else?

I told her. She followed me around as I helped to get the breakfast ready, pursuing the matter. An hour later she was going home for the weekend and she sought me out as she went.

Martine   You've told me all the bad things about myself. Isn't there a single good thing you could say?

Merely manipulative? If so, I was manipulated. From that point onwards I saw a human being with human needs in Martine. Much later, when we met again on another ward she said one day 'Oh Margaret, I do wish I weren't like this.' Insincere? I thought not.

Take other illnesses. Although 'I can't help being like this, I am a schizophrenic' can be used to the speaker's advantage, it can be frightening when used by others. 'Don't employ him, he's a schizophrenic.' 'You don't want to get involved with her, she's a schizophrenic.' Or 'she's an epileptic.'

Whereas really these people are Martine, John, Tina, June. People with problems that are bad enough to bear in themselves, without the labels adding yet more burdens by further preventing the development of normal relationships with others.

If we have managed to identify the problem exactly, if we have got our labelling right, the danger is that we stop seeing the people behind that label.

And I must not finish this section on the danger of fixing firm diagnoses without spelling out again something I first discussed while writing about roles.

Knowing one's diagnosis can undoubtedly be helpful to a patient. 'I am a schizophrenic.' 'I am a manic-depressive.' 'I am an agoraphobic.' 'I am an anorexic.' In other words: 'This terrible thing that so handicaps and frightens me is not unique to me. There are many other people who suffer similarly and I stand a good chance of getting some help from what the doctors have learnt in the past from them and from treatments that have already been tried. Knowing what is the matter with me and being able to talk to my fellow-sufferers and being able to read about them makes me feel less isolated and helpless.' All this is good.

Nevertheless there is a danger in 'I am a . . .'. It can carry the spoken or unspoken addition 'and there is nothing I can do about it. This is how I am and how I will remain.'

Look at some physical parallels - blind people, lame, deaf. 1981 was the 'Year of the Disabled'. A man in a wheelchair, addressing a meeting, explained the difference between a disability and a handicap in his eyes: 'A disability is a fact. I am disabled in that I cannot walk. But the extent to which it is a handicap is up to me. I have a severe handicap if I allow my disability to rule my life.' The speaker did not see himself primarily as 'a man in a wheelchair'.

So with schizophrenia and manic-depression, agoraphobia, anorexia and all the other psychiatric problems. There is no doubt that these are disabilities, as it is for men and women in wheelchairs. But 'I am a . . . ' is dangerous. 'I am *me!*' is important. With everything that makes me *me,* and especially with all the positives: 'I enjoy writing letters. I can cook a reasonable meal. I have a cheerful grin.'

Let's make good uses of diagnoses when we can. And let's also recognise the dangers and avoid them, both as outsiders and as sufferers.

THE DIFFICULTY OF BEING SURE

The consultant who lectured to us on mental illnesses taught us Ockam's law: 'Causes should not be unnecessarily multiplied'. That was true, said the consultant, of general medicine, where a single cause might explain a complicated picture, but it was not true of psychiatry.

So, take Michael. We know he had a disturbed childhood. A father in the theatre, whose work was spasmodic, sometimes working intensely hard and away and unable to see his son, and sometimes not working at all and spending much time with him. That father left the family when Michael was nine years old, and he was the eldest of four children in a fatherless home. He became involved at one time with a drug-taking set, and we still do not know what he took and whether that physically damaged him. The national employment crisis meant that so many of his contemporaries were unemployed. And - aha - it later turned out that his grandmother had been, for a time anyway, bizarrely ill and in a mental hospital.

A multiplicity of possible causes. And what does it make Michael in terms of a diagnosis? He is not obviously deluded or hallucinated. He comes across so warmly. (Or does he really? He smiles a lot, but is it real warmth?) Surely he is not a schizophrenic? Surely he could help himself a lot more? Is he merely lazy? It is very difficult indeed to be properly objective about Michael. At 26 his life is beginning to slip tragically by. Whatever is wrong? Surely we should be able to help? But how?

That last paragraph was written while standing in the nurses' shoes. Let's step into Michael's: 'You can't keep me here. Why? What have I done? I'm not ill.' But at other times: 'I need help. I can't concentrate. I have these obsessive thoughts. You've got to help.'

We could pin almost any label on Michael: neurotic, psychotic, behavioural problem, schizophrenia, obsessional disorder, depression. Diagnosing Michael seems almost impossible. And while we have already helped him we still haven't found a complete cure.

DIAGNOSING - AN EMOTIVE SUBJECT

I had written this chapter thus far when a personal experience brought me up with a jolt. At the time a nursing journal was carrying a 16-week series of pieces by me: 'A Psychiatric Sister's ABC' (Putnam, 1981). Under D for Diagnosis I had briefly spelled out the difficulties of being sure 'what some patients were' and the importance of seeing them primarily as themselves, as individuals whose individuality we wished to retain and allow to develop further. I had thought that fair and kind.

To my astonishment our hospital's legal expert sought me out to tell me how a letter had arrived which had had some of the hospital's senior staff in a state of alarm. It was an angry letter - requesting my dismissal! - from a woman in another part of the country who had personally found it very helpful and important to her to know that she was schizophrenic and who was horrified at the idea that nurses might withold a diagnosis from a patient.

I could see at once a parallel from general medicine and from my own experience. I had had a series of lumps in my breast over many years. My first was at 23. The consultant of that time, trying to be kind, had been too quick with his reassurance that it would not be cancer, so that when I had a second lump at 27 I was convinced that the first had been malignant and that the second was a recurrence. As a mother with two small sons that was terrifying. And maybe it was my open terror that made the doctors in my new area so straight with me. Their willingness to let me ask questions and their open answers about the second lump, a genuine cancer this time, was extraordinarily helpful, and here I am now, more than 20 years and two more breast lumps (both innocent) later, quite able to cope with the subject.

So, I could appreciate the wrath of the schizophrenic who felt angry that I might wish to cover up a diagnosis of schizophrenia and prevent helpful discussion.

I can fully see from my own illness how frightening a cover-up attitude is. Covering-up suggests that there are terrible truths best not known. That certainly is not an attitude I would encourage - quite the reverse.

The point is that it must be the truth that we pass on. And, as yet, it frequently appears to be difficult to be sure what the truth is. So, if we have to say something, it must be 'We don't properly know what is wrong, and we can't be sure how to help.' This must be very frightening to people who want answers and a promise of help.

It has sometimes seemed to me that we have come full circle:

from groping to groping. That once there was little knowledge of the mental illnesses, and that gradually a vast amount of material was gathered and sorted and the illnesses classified, and that now there is so much debate again on some topics that we wonder whether we know anything at all. I am sure we do. I am sure, also, that it is good for us to remind ourselves that there is very much more still to learn.

So it does seem wise to very many of us working in the psychiatric sphere not to slap too firm a diagnosis too readily on a patient. We look back through patients' files and see 'schizophrenia' again and again. It looks so much as if the policy once was, 'When in doubt diagnose schizophrenia.' So now we hesitate. OK, there is something strange about Derek, John, Adrian, Roger, Patsy, Mavis, Linda, etc., etc. They laugh to themselves weirdly at times, they have difficulty in getting on with other people, they are restless and cannot settle in work, they are extremely bothering to us because something is very clearly wrong and yet there seems no clear-cut way to put it right. But are they schizophrenic?

And, very often, they are young. In their twenties, and it seems desperately important that whatever is wrong should be put right before it is too late and they are stuck with their inability to live life to the full.

Emotive, I said, and I'll own up. I find it difficult as a psychiatric nurse to stay wholly detached at all times.

But having said that, I'll say this too: that I am not wholly overinvolved either. The golden mean has got to apply! While I am very concerned for the young patients that we seem unable to help, I realise how essential it is that once off-duty I recharge my batteries by living my own personal life fully before the next span of duty and the next round of drain upon my emotional, mental and physical energy.

But this is the main point I wish to make here: If nurses and doctors and others who work in the psychiatric sphere really care about the people we so often seem so powerless to help, how do those people themselves feel, and their relatives?

Trying to be sure what is wrong and trying to see how to put it right inevitably arouses emotions. It must be a very cold person indeed who imagines that everyone can stay at all times completely objective about it!

Diagnosis and the Schizophrenia Debate

WHAT IS SCHIZOPHRENIA?

In the last section, I told how I distressed someone by saying I was reluctant to talk very certainly about our patients' schizophrenia to our nurses. And that person's distress has made me question the wisdom of including this section in this book. But I will, first reiterating that it is one nurse's view only, and that it includes a large number of questions which I see as important but to which I do not know the answers. It cannot be my very honest book if I omit my views and my questions about schizophrenia, especially as these views and questions are held and asked by others too.

The first question is: does schizophrenia really exist? Bleuler coined the term 'the schizophrenias', a group of closely related illnesses, or an illness with variations (and which way he saw it does not matter too much here). Kraepelin had, a little earlier, decided that many of the patients in the mental hospitals were not individually and uniquely mad but that their similar symptoms suggested an illness that could be identified and studied (Mayer-Gross *et al.*, 1954).

Kraepelin and Bleuler had their opponents who disbelieved their findings. So, second question: who was right - Kraepelin and Bleuler in identifying the illness or the others in disputing their findings? Dispute was probably inevitable; it accompanies most major discoveries.

One of my ideas that allows me to think Kraepelin and Bleuler just may have been in error is that many of the symptoms of schizophrenia as we see them within the hospitals - and it was from in-patients that Kraepelin first made his deductions - could be the result of the patients' long stay in an institution, the asylum of Kraepelin's day, the psychiatric hospital of today. Putting myself into the shoes of a long-stay patient I can well imagine myself becoming apathetic about the day-by-day existence in hospital, becoming withdrawn and disorganised, building a dream world in preference to my surroundings, and often appearing bizarre in my words and deeds.

It is all very debatable. I can at once pick holes in my own ideas. If I built a dream world would it develop the frightening aspects of the delusions and hallucinations of many patients? (But, then, I think it might.) What of the acute schizophrenic illness that starts outside the hospital? That is not a result of institutionalisation.

However, I would not dare to ask 'Does schizophrenia exist?' in my own right. I was first taught to do so by a former consultant of mine who when nurses talked very readily about schizophrenia would flummox them by saying 'Ah, schizophrenia - what is that?' Gradually I learnt a little about the views of R.D. Laing (1960) and Thomas S. Szasz (1962), and I discovered from them that schizophrenia was a debatable subject.

My present view is that it may well exist as a genuine illness, but we must be careful not to use the term too readily. And we do need to know what we are meaning by the term.

The next important question is: if schizophrenia exists, how is it caused?

Is it caused by chemical imbalance, by excessive dopamine and other chemically wrong levels in the synapse area between certain brain nerve transmitters and receptors? Or is there a physical abnormality in that certain nerve receptors are over-finely tuned and respond in an exaggerated fashion? Or is it both a chemical and physical malfunction? Obviously there is a very great deal of research into schizophrenia, and this research does suggest such malfunctions (Hemmings, 1982).

Many people, myself included, feel that the schizophrenic symptoms may also result from an inability to cope with life as the patient finds it. We can look at the lives of some schizophrenic patients and say, with hindsight, 'Yes, that could well have been very distressing . . . Yes, of course that must have made her feel very insecure.' So, further questions: Can a distressing early life, or a sufficiently traumatic later life, in itself trigger off a schizophrenic illness? And if so, how? If some schizophrenics have a genetic chemical imbalance, do others develop a similar imbalance through their particular reactions to extreme stress? Or do they develop similar symptoms without any chemical malfunctioning? And are there a larger number of potential schizophrenics with mild genetic chemical imbalance who never develop the distressing symptoms because they have grown up in particularly stable and suitable-to-them homes and have never been exposed to situations they found intolerable?

I add that 'suitable-to-them' because I am so convinced of our individuality. One person's stable background is another's unbearable boredom; one person's adventurousness and flexibility is another's insecurity.

If this is read by the person I angered so much previously, it will certainly anger her yet again, and understandably so. In my 'Psychiatric Sister's ABC' I did not suggest that schizophrenia may not exist. She is a schizophrenic sufferer and knows better than any nurse all that that means to her. Of course it exists, she and her fellow sufferers must say.

What I am trying to say, and I do not find it easy to write this in a crystal-clear fashion because it does not seem to be a crystal-clear matter, is that the term 'schizophrenia' was once used far too readily, and that we now need to know what we mean when we use that term.

To summarise: are we now able to say that there is an organic cause that gives rise to the symptoms that Kraepelin and Bleuler recognised as frequently combining into this illness? Is it genetic? (And that must lead to further questions about heredity, not attempted here, although I know that it has been studied (Mayer-Gross *et al.*, 1954).) Can the organic malfunction be triggered off by stress? Can stress produce in some people the same set of symptoms independently, without organic malfunction?

We do not have clear enough answers yet to these questions. This is distressing, and is one reason why this section is taking so much space. The patients and their relatives badly want clear answers. They look to the doctors and nurses to provide those answers, and few of us feel confident enough to give very definite answers.

There are a large number of patients whose 'schizophrenia' is fiercely debated by their staff. They present many of the symptoms: hallucinations, delusions, lack of concentration, a frequent lack of drive, difficulty in forming and keeping stable relationships. And yet the nurses have a strong sense of 'This is not a schizophrenic patient.'

Take Derek. When he was transferred to my ward I looked in

astonishment at a recent nursing note: 'Derek has not been biting people's ankles so much lately.' I gathered he talked often of his 'voices'. And yet I felt instinctively that he was not schizophrenic. Rightly or wrongly, I persuaded Derek that he was not basically 'ill' but that he had problems in coping with everyday life.

'Those voices you get', I said (not sticking my neck right out and saying 'You don't have voices') 'are linked to your feeling stressed. Try to get out of the habit of talking so much about your voices. Try to tell us that you are feeling particularly stressed.'

His outward presentation at least became a great deal more normal. Derek is still in hospital more than a year later, but no longer on my ward. A new consultant gathered together a group of these 'What are they really?' patients.

I wondered at one point about doing some research into these patients. What was really the matter? They were often young. They talked readily about their voices to anyone and everyone - whereas those I would describe as more obviously schizophrenic seldom do. They persuaded their doctors into changing their medication frequently, trying first this and then that, tranquillisers, antidepressants, anxiolytics, the long tried as well as the latest on the market. It seemed so often that they could not properly cope with life and found an escape and support in the psychiatric hospital to which they repeatedly returned, despite the staff's feeling that they should be able to cope outside. But when I looked up 'inadequate' in the *Cumulated Index Medicus* I found 'Inadequate personality - see Personality disorder', which brings us closer to 'psychopaths'.

Another question: what then is a psychopath? No! I am not going to become embroiled in that one here! The point is, between the recognisable schizophrenic and the undoubted psychopath lies a great grey area, a very large number of people who need help but whose diagnoses cannot exactly be determined.

Finally, back to Derek. I was talking to his new consultant over a hospital meal. We both liked Derek. We talked fast and happily about him even though it was our break.

He You know, I have a feeling he may be really schizophrenic after all. There is something a degree odd about him, I think.

Me Really? Well, yes, perhaps you're right.

OTHER DEBATABLE ILLNESSES

In the area where I now work, a rehabilitation/medium-/long-stay ward (that it, we like to think that all our ward's patients may go back into the community somehow one day, though some have already been in the hospital for decades), it is the schizophrenia-inadequate-behavioural debate that looms above all others. So when I was asked whether I was getting it out of proportion in writing a separate section on it, my first reaction was of astonishment at the question, and my second reaction was a confident 'No!'

But, taking a more objective view, I realise that many illnesses are not instantly and certainly diagnosed. Not even in the general hospital.

In the psychiatric field on an acute ward I have heard staff debating whether certain anorexic young ladies were suffering from a clear-cut 'illness', or whether they were 'acting-out' in refusing to eat and were almost 'psychopathic'.

On my present ward too one patient in particular dominated the scene for a long time. We never ever thought she was schizophrenic. That was the one certain thing on which everyone agreed. And we all agreed that she had a severe behavioural problem. In her case the debate was whether she could also be called a genuine manic-depressive.

So what?

DOES IT MATTER IF THE DIAGNOSIS IS HARD TO MAKE?

So what?

This is not a rude comment. It is an extremely important question. Is it vitally important that a psychiatric illness shall be clearly diagnosed? What effect does it have on people if it is difficult to be certain?

As I am a nurse I wish to speak first from the nurses'

viewpoint. It can be very disruptive if some nurses feel strongly that a difficult patient is 'almost psychopathic' while others feel equally strongly that he/she is 'schizophrenic'.

The truth is that, whatever patients are, they need help of some sort! Most patients need help to discover how best to help themselves, how best to get themselves, the world and life into better perspective. Very many people need this help - nurses and other professionals, too, very often, and not just our patients!

There often seems to remain in psychiatric hospitals a belief that people with behavioural problems, that is, not an organic illness, really could in the last resort pull themselves together if only they would make a superhuman effort. In fact, some nurses seem to feel that certain patients could pull themselves together very easily, while the truly 'ill' patients may be excused a great deal. The nurses too can take the line 'He is a schizophrenic/manic depressive . . . She is anorexic/agoraphobic. They cannot help themselves.'

What follows from such thinking is this: the patients we find it easy to like are 'ill schizophrenics', whereas the patients we find it hard to like are 'manipulating people who could change if only they didn't so much enjoy making trouble for others'. And given such a rift between the staff, the next stage is that, for example, the nurses will be saying to each other:

'You only say So-and-so is schizophrenic because you like her.'

'You only say So-and-so is psychopathic because you don't like her.'

This is a destructive atmosphere. Bad for both the nurses and for the patients. The patients cannot be helped in such an atmosphere.

So, let's look at the effects on the patients if their diagnosis is not wholly clear.

One, alas, that follows on from what has been said above is that nurses who feel the patient chooses to behave badly will tend to treat the patients poorly. This could even mean the patient may be rough-handled physically. It has occasionally happened - items have reached newspapers, inquiries have been set up and reports subsequently published (for example, SE Thames RHA, 1976). Such unacceptable staff behaviour has been well exposed in *Conscientious Objectors at work* (Beardshaw, 1981).

But almost equally bad, in my view, is the day-by-day awareness that one is disliked. Put yourself in the shoes of a patient for whom the hospital is 'home', where the people with most authority, the staff, make it very clear that they would rather you were not here. I wrote in an earlier chapter about Martine, whom I myself had disliked. Gradually I came to understand how it might feel to be disliked. To have one set of nurses that disliked me going off duty to their homes and their families for them only to be replaced by another set who disliked me equally. To have no home or family to which I could myself leave, because I was somehow lumbered with a bloody-minded nature which I felt powerless to change. From time to time I - Martine - say 'I wish I weren't like this!' but I know that the nurses don't believe me.

And now I admit that I am right back to questions of the staff's attitudes to patients, which is where this book started.

That can't be helped. The diagnoses and our attitudes to patients are closely intermingled, and all those who work in psychiatric hospitals need to recognise that.

References

Arieti, S. (1978). On schizophrenia, phobias, depression, psychotherapy and the farther shores of psychiatry, *Selected Papers of Silvano Arieti*, New York: Brunner and Mazel.

Beardshaw, V. (1981). *Conscientious Objectors at Work*, London: Social Audit.

Hemmings, G. (1982). *Biological Aspects of Schizophrenia and Addiction*, Chichester: John Wiley.

Laing, R.D. (1960). *The Divided Self*, London: Tavistock Publications.

Mayer-Gross, W., Slater, E. and Roth, M. (1954). *Clinical Psychiatry*, London: Ballière, Tindall and Cassell. (For references to Kraepelin and Bleuler.)

Putnam, M. (1981). 'A Psychiatric Sister's ABC', *The Nursing Times*, 5 March - 17 June (16-week series).

SE Thames RHA (1976). *Report of Committee of Inquiry, St Augustine's Hospital, Chatham, Canterbury,* South East Thames Regional Health Authority.

Szasz, T.S. (1962). *The Myth of Mental Illness,* London: Secker and Warburg. (Also 1972, St Albans: Paladin.)

5 Patients and Treatments

So Many Ways to Try

Over and over in my few years as a psychiatric nurse, and especially during my four years as a sister, I have been appalled by my lack of knowledge. I have been aware too that there are great areas in which I could study much more and don't. Why haven't I explored my own subject very much more?

Partly because there is so much! Where on earth are we to start? The nursing journals come out week by week, and though I take one regularly and sometimes two, I don't always read them. I have failed to read much more partly because, despite the wordage, there seems to be so much debate still. Unless the time spent on reading and studying truly helps me to help others - and I am not sure it will - I can better use that time.

Those who are working closely with psychiatric patients need to get totally away for large periods of time. This is often not properly appreciated, even by those who in their time have worked very closely with patients. 'Nurses don't read!' complains an excellent tutor who reads a lot. 'Yes, I do', I reply. 'Lots of novels.' And to digress one degree: that may not be so far from the job either. One consultant said he wished nurses would spend less time reading psychology textbooks and more time reading good novels about people and the way they ticked, alone and in their relationships.

Relationships - this book keeps returning to them.

But first I will try to produce a random list of the ways in which we might try to help our psychiatric patients.

ECT	Deconditioning
Drugs	Narcosis
Abreaction	Psychotherapy groups
Work regimes	Token economy methods
Hypnosis	Therapeutic community
Leucotomy (modern forms)	methods

Counselling	Individual care programmes
Psychoanalysis	Nursing process techniques
Behaviour therapy	Drama therapy
Social skills training	Food-allergy studies
	(Mackarness, 1976)

However, I was in Zambia a little while ago, and was staying on the campus of the country's only psychiatric hospital.

Me (to pupil nurse) What do you think is the most important kind of help we can give to the patients? Out of all the range of treatments what will help them most?

Nurse (after a pause) Building a good rapport with them.

Me Hurrah! Come back and work with me in Britain! No! On second thoughts, you are needed here too!

I wondered, 'Can young Zambians thought-read?' I must explain that this was a spur of the moment question in an informal discussion as I was being shown around. The previous part of the conversation had not obviously led up to that answer.

I have explained earlier that this book is one nurse's view, and not an authoritative book giving known and undebatable facts. And here now I will permit myself to speak up loudly on topics that are personal and exceedingly debatable.

I was in Zambia for three weeks. In my absence the 'rule-makers' on my ward appear to have had more sway! To my mind 'rule' is a dirty word, whereas 'routine' I approve of. A routine is a helpful pattern, a general guide, so that we don't have to think out every action. Routines are evolved to suit everyone, staff and patients alike, and are adapted as needed from time to time. But 'rules' carry more than a hint of inflexibility, and they tend to be imposed by the staff on the patients.

Patients like routines: 'What day is my depot injection?' 'Breakfast is late today, isn't it?' 'I like to go to bed early.' 'I like to go to bed late.' In fact, there must be variation in the routines of individual patients. But the rules so often work against the patients, and they are so often imposed on everyone because of the undesirable behaviour of a few!

I find that in my absence these rules have raised their heads more positively. Rules about not lying on beds, about not wearing dressing gowns to breakfast, about not allowing cups of tea to patients from other wards. That's another aspect of rules - they are so often prohibitive.

I wrote earlier about the ward meetings we have been having in recent months. So often, it seems to be me on duty for the Wednesday afternoon ward meeting! I certainly had not done the duty rota for my first week back from Zambia, but it was me who was leading the ward meeting yet again. I am a great chatterer, but I do know how to pick out and give a space to everyone who is bursting with something to say in those meetings. And plenty of these patients had plenty to say at the ward meeting when I got back about the restrictions and the change of staff attitudes and the oppression, as they saw it. It was embarrassing anyway. We must work as a staff team. It was extra embarrassing in that we had a visitor from much higher in the hospital's hierarchy. But she is, I gather, a wise woman and knew that nurses tend to fall into two groups, those who see discipline as a highly important part of helping people, and those who appear to be more easy-going. She joined in my assurance that those who had lately appeared to be somewhat oppressive were working entirely for the patients' good and with the best of intentions.

I put all this down, though it is so specific to me and my ward at this time (although it must be echoed all over this country and other countries), because it is so relevant to 'building a good rapport'.

We need to go back to that golden mean. Of course the patients should not be lying on their beds the whole day and every day - and one or two of my patients almost do that. Of course they should not appear at breakfast ill-clad and dishevelled. Of course our 'household' must not be imposed upon by other patients whose only interest in us is the free cup of tea. But we must not counteract one bad with another bad! We must not swing from one extreme to the other.

I am writing close to these events. If I am too far distanced from my experiences I both forget them and become too lazy to write about them. It is what the patients and the staff are saying today that I keep noting. Psychiatric nursing is so much an on-going thing. We must never assume that by now we know it all. We must keep listening and keep thinking about what we hear.

This I maintain - under every method there must be a rapport between the helper and the helped. I will not say 'between the nurse and the patient'. While I am proud to say 'I am a psychiatric nurse', because I love my work and I love talking about it, in reality I see myself as a person with people. Others besides the nurses will also help. See the next chapter about the hospital staff, and the following one about the patients' relatives, and beyond that for those who help in the community. Basically, it will be their rapport, their ability to relate well, that makes the helpers able to help, whatever the way they are trying.

PS: At the end of yesterday's ward meeting, which had lasted over the allotted hour, we realised we had done nothing except work our way through the points arising from the previous minutes.

Me   I think we should stop. But is there anything else

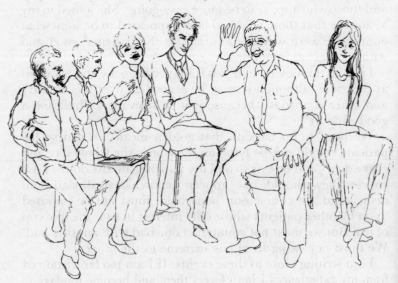

that anyone is bursting to say? Anything that can't wait till next week?

Kevin May I suggest that we have a day when we patients run the ward, and the staff act as the patients?

This caused much delight. Several patients began at once, all talking together, to explain the treatment they would give the staff. This stage of the meeting was entirely good-humoured. There is a good rapport here mostly. But could the patients have said any more openly: 'Please put yourself in our shoes'?

The Patient Receiving Treatment

If there were just one point to be made in this book, it would have to be 'put yourself constantly into the patients' shoes, again and again, under differing circumstances. Ask yourself "How would I feel if this were me?" '

I was listening to a patient's mother on the phone. The conversation had taken an unexpected turn.

Mother . . . and I don't approve of this business of making the patients cry.

Me (in utter bewilderment) Making the patients cry? No-one here sets out to make anyone cry - not to my knowledge, at least. I know Patricia does cry quite a bit, but that isn't part of her treatment!

Mother Oh. I thought perhaps it was. I think it used to be.

Patricia was once a day-patient in a group that included drama therapy. I myself had recently attended a co-counselling training week and had found myself crying, to my amazement and to my relief. Although I know myself to be an emotional person, I keep my unhappiness and my anger to myself as much as I can, disliking effusive displays of emotion in others, and not wishing to annoy or embarrass others by any displays of my own. I put all this down here, in order to say that we do need to consider what it is we are doing in our treatment, what effect it is having, and whether the overall benefit is helpful or harmful.

I still do not know whether Patricia was ever 'made to cry'. I keep meaning to ask her about this, but it is not particularly relevant to Patricia at the moment and a thousand other matters intrude between us and that interesting conversation piece.

Instead let's take the more common ECT, modified electro-convulsive therapy, and the use of drugs, both of which I know more about.

Not that I have much experience of ECT now. It is practically never used on my ward. It is used far more with the acutely ill patients. But Andrew, who has not long transferred to us from an acute ward, seemed so severely depressed that the consultant saw this as the only way of lifting him. Andrew was very apprehensive. He had never had ECT. So a sensitive student nurse began explaining to him exactly what was involved, trying to guess the erroneous imaginings that Andrew might have. Andrew would not feel any shock at all, he told him. He would have an anaesthetic to put him to sleep for the brief period of the treatment. The student went on to explain that the patient is not 'wired up', and that a current is applied for the briefest of time only. 'It is rather like touching an electric fence. Have you ever done that, Andrew?'

As so often, I learnt myself from this occasion. I was still present with Andrew and the nurse when Margery came looking for that nurse.

Me Can you wait a moment, Margery? Phil is telling Andrew about ECT. Dr Smith thinks Andrew might be helped out of his low mood by it, but Andrew is anxious about it.

Margery (turning to Andrew) Oh, you don't need to be! You won't feel a thing. I've had it a lot in the past and it really helped me.

That surprised me. I hadn't thought of patients reassuring patients about ECT. Perhaps in my student days when I was present at ECT sessions I had known that this was possible, but if so I had forgotten it.

Andrew agreed to have it, but remained unhappy about it. We watched Andrew through his first, second, third sessions.

The course was half-way through and had he improved? Possibly our anxiety rubbed off on to Andrew. He himself began to debate whether it was helping him. He seemed to have listened now to other patients who talked of ECT leaving people with damaged brains.

'I don't want to have any more ECT', Andrew began saying. 'It can leave you brain-damaged.'

What was a good nurse to do? And, especially, what were good nurses to do who themselves wondered about the effect of ECT on the brain?

What would you have said? Pause and think, and then see if it is anything like our conversation.

Nurse There is debate about ECT, Andrew. Some people do think it can cause damage if used too often. But we have millions of brain cells. Three more sessions of ECT will cause only the absolutely microscopic amount of damage, if any. And it could help a very great deal.

Andrew (laughing - though clearly it was rueful laughter) I don't want even one or two of those brain cells damaged, thank you.

Nurse But you don't want to stay so very depressed either, do you? In fact, you are probably already somewhat better. We couldn't have had so reasonable or cheerful a conversation as this two weeks ago.

Andrew Perhaps I am a bit better.

Nurse Compromise. Finish this course of six ECTs. Anything less than that will probably not help you as much as you need. But when you have had the course of six sessions, *then* if you feel very strongly against ECT still, we will back you up. It is true you don't have to have any more now. We can't make you. But we can advise you to try these six.

And that was what happened. Andrew completed the course. By then he had come out of his utter dejection and the consultant was happy to leave the course at the set of six sessions.

Also, Andrew was accompanied to the sessions by a nurse

who liked Andrew and who was liked by Andrew. The same nurse went with him each time, as far as was possible.

Such individual treatment, with a one-to-one nurse-patient involvement, is not possible on an acute ward where several patients are having ECT at each session. The outstanding fact to me, when I was a student regularly involved in ECT in the acute area, was that the most important place for an understanding nurse to be was not the treatment room itself so much as the waiting room. And, next in importance, someone sensitive should be with the patients after the treatment is all over. ECT is not, with rare exceptions, a treatment that patients like. Painless though it is, it causes apprehension beforehand and confusion afterwards. Put yourself in the patients' shoes. Both before and after ECT the patient needs the cheerful, sensitive support of imaginative nurses.

As for patients and their drugs! Where does one begin on this discussion?

Patients want to know about their drugs. 'What is this for?' 'What will it do?' 'How soon will it work?' They are not wholly sure that they want it.

This reminds me of an experience of a nursing friend. She was giving a patient her much needed anticoagulant. (When talking about our psychiatric drugs to the student nurses from the general hospital I begin by explaining that we also have a wide range of physical drugs in our trolleys.)

Nurse   Here is your wayfarin, Mrs Jones.
Another patient (leaping out of the queue)   Don't take it, Mary! That is rat poison!

Yes, a very alarming drug name to the patient who overheard. A paranoid patient perhaps, already suspicious about the treatments being offered!

How is one to help the patients who do not want their medications?

Maybe the astonishing thing is that the patients are as compliant as they are - although their compliance of course does not mean that the drugs are always taken! Psychiatric hospitals all have their stories. There was the geriatric chair that spilled out its tubeful of tablets when upended in a ward move. The chair's regular user, a sweet little old lady, had systematically popped them into the slot intended for the chair's table. There was the middle-aged patient about to go to a group home who owned up that she would not need the drugs she had 'been having' for years. She had always thrown them down the lift shaft with no ill effect to herself.

But back to the question: what are we to do when the patient refuses medication? The answers must vary. The patients are individuals. Why is the patient refusing? Has he/she any valid reason? One patient pinned me against a wall once when I discovered she was dropping her tablets into her skirt. She loathed the taste so much and she was petrified, she explained afterwards, that I'd ram them down her throat. The awful part of that experience to me was not the brief fear of an attack, but the discovery that she could imagine I might force tablets into her. I won her over by, first, not holding her reaction against her; secondly, sucking one of the tablets myself and discovering that it did indeed have a nasty taste if not swallowed quickly; and thirdly, being able to obtain an alternative for her which she was willing to take.

The message of all this piece is: Do listen to the patients. Listen to their physical complaints about their medication. And observe them. It wasn't until one patient flaked out for the second time within a day or two that a thoughtful nurse said 'Could it be that tricyclic? Doesn't that also reduce the blood pressure? Look at her admission notes. Her blood pressure was already on the low side then, wasn't it?'

Back to that argumentative ward meeting I mentioned earlier. The patients insisted then, as they had insisted before, that they lie on their beds because they feel very tired. 'It's the tranquillisers', a lot of them said. It may be. John, an angry young man at times, said 'It's quite ridiculous. I wake up feeling knocked out, and then you come round with the drug trolley and say "It's time you were up, John. Here's your tranquilliser." '

It was ridiculous. We cut down the tranquillisers and altered the times at which the remainder was given. And we put the responsibility for his behaviour back on to John himself: 'You are right, John. You probably need less medication. Show us you are right by not allowing yourself to lose your temper so readily.'

'OK', said John, and he has done that.

I am glad John is an angry young man, even though our relationship is often uncomfortable. The too compliant long-stay patients are probably unbudgeable from the hospital now. John takes a more active part in his own treatment.

Two urgent points need to be made about drug use and abuse. First, let's keep alert and be absolutely sure as we give out the medications that the patients really do need all these tablets. I certainly don't mean that we should withold every second one, tossing a coin as it were - 'Shall we give this one or not?' 'Shall we give that one or not?' The drugs were prescribed originally for a purpose. But we do need to ask ourselves if the purpose still holds and if the original strength of the tablet is still needed. We need to keep reviewing the drugs with the doctors.

Second point: This is another time to apply the golden mean. Let's not swing to either extreme. Drugs are not perfect and unique cure-alls. We cannot say in every case 'The patient has such and such an illness and drug X will cure it.' But nor should we totally abandon all psychiatric drugs because it is realised that there are side-effects. We should be aiming rather for an ideal balance. We must weigh the original severe mental distress against a present, as-slight-as-possible drug-caused problem. We must not lose our sense of proportion.

Some nurses have at times annoyed, and deep down upset, me by harping on about the old pre-Largactil era and how they had to 'do proper psychiatric nursing then'. But there was truth in their comment. The points they were making were that until the mid 1950s there were far fewer tranquillisers; the patients' moods were far less predictable; controlling the patients was a major part of the nurses' task.

We need to remind ourselves of this from time to time. On the whole the general public has little idea, I believe, how reasonable psychiatric patients are now. The old image remains of patients who are screaming and violent, at least at times; and of nurses whose job consists primarily in controlling their patients' moods. Nurses and others working in psychiatric hospitals can help to explain that our patients are very very rarely like that, and, if our patients are out and about as much as they should be, they themselves will be showing that they are not so extreme. But also, we must remember that for many of our patients it is the tranquillisers that help initially by reducing their disturbance so that we can then go on to helping them to build the better relationships that in turn keep them more stable.

That is almost certainly oversimplifying again. On my ward we have 30 patients and I am daily astonished at their individuality.

This section is called 'The patient receiving treatment'. Don't we need to be reminding ourselves constantly how individual that treatment needs to be? And alas, I have spoken far too much about drugs here and little else, and that is because the drugs do still play an unreasonably high part in patient care in very many wards - including my own.

The Patient as Part of the Team

These two chapters about the patients' diagnoses and treatments are difficult to write. I want to stop and review how far we have got:

It is important to listen to what the patients feel about their treatments.

One of the questions put to me at my interview when I first became a ward sister was, 'Who do you think should be involved in discussions about patients?' I began my answer with, 'The patient first of all.' Now after several years as a sister I stand by that. I hope this book so far has shown that it is my practice to talk *with* patients far more than *about* patients.

This is the ideal then: involving the patients. Talking with them. Listening to them. Hearing their experiences. Hearing what they feel might help them most - and in very many cases their illness has lasted decades and they have had a great variety of treatments and drugs, and they know what they feel to be the most helpful.

Of course the patient and the rest of the multidisciplinary team may not agree on the best course of action. Recently Jack was abnormally disturbed. He was having a love problem. The young lady who had taken his fancy did not fancy him. It upset him so much that it put him right off work - and he had been going out to work from the hospital for over a year. He marched around smashing three or four cups and a plate or two and tearing notices off the board, all the time keeping an eye on us and making sure that we were noticing this. We handled this as well as we could, mainly with large doses of sympathy: 'Poor old Jack, it's rotten, we know.'

But this seemed a time for extra tranquilliser. 'Would you let us give you some extra tranquilliser? You could even have a long sleep today and see if that helps a bit, eh?'

Jack shook his head. He is a silent man. A strong and silent man. When a doctor tried to overrule Jack and said that a change of medication was a must, Jack looked for the biggest book he could find, the ward's diary-cum-handover book, and began tearing it into two.

'Oh dear', said the doctor.

Jack made his point, which we already knew: that over the years he has found his present medication absolutely ideal, and it is on this that he has improved to the point of living so nearly normal a life that he is now able to bank a goodly sum each week with a view to living outside again one day.

Jack was lucky. Not all patients get as good a hearing, though hearing is not quite the word, for few words were exchanged. With a different sister and a different doctor Jack's method of saying 'I don't agree with you and I don't wish to have the treatment you are proposing' might have convinced his observers that they were right and Jack was wrong, and he might have had the extra tranquilliser willy-nilly. Instead we both said, 'OK, Jack, you've made your point! But if tranquillisers won't help you, nor will smashing the cups really. We don't want to run out of them. What will the others do without cups?'

I am not sure we do listen to the patients enough yet.

And lest I make all this sound all very simple - of course it is not! That episode with Jack put the ward staff under a lot of strain. Were we handling his aggression correctly? At present he was venting his wrath on things, but might he turn it upon his fellow-patients or upon a member of staff? I did not want anyone hurt. But nor did I want Jack upset any more than he already was. Handle Jack wrongly and his great improvement might have been totally lost.

Jack did not speak much, but when patients do express themselves volubly it is not always easy to understand what they are saying. Or is it that when patients express some of their ideas somewhat bizarrely we fail to realise how much to the point many of their comments are? I think in particular of one young lady, Lesley, who seemed so strange. Most of the nurses, even the trained psychiatric nurses, said 'What a load of rubbish Lesley talks!' It was a cheerful extroverted general nurse on a mere eight weeks experience with us who told me one evening how grieved she was about Lesley. 'She tells us all the time how unhappy she is, and how desolate, and how apprehensive she is about her future doesn't she!' I was glad to find someone else who realised how clearly Lesley spelled out her feelings again and again in her own manner.

Not that listening and hearing enabled us to help Lesley much. She was herself convinced that little could be done to help her, and though she came to us often and talked a lot she seldom stayed for our answers. But it did help her just a bit to know that some of us understood how she felt.

Fortunately Lesley was an extreme. Most patients who sit in multidisciplinary meetings with the consultant, a doctor or two, the social worker, nurses, occupational therapist, and perhaps a relative, can explain themselves better and can contribute to their own futures.

Learning to Live With the Problem

I have never forgotten that consultant, mentioned much earlier, who replied to the comment, 'Celia's heaps better', by asking, 'Are you sure better is the right word?'

These two chapters have been hard to write because they are about the patients' diagnoses and treatments, that is, their 'illnesses'. 'Illnesses' is still how we see it all. And 'illnesses' implies 'cures'.

I have used a great deal of space explaining that it is often far from easy to be sure exactly what is wrong. And since beginning on this topic I have had a new patient on my ward, Linda. She shouldn't be on our ward at all. She has come to us sheerly because the acute wards have no empty beds and because her home situation has become intolerable. She has obsessional fears about germs. Linda can understand and explain her problem and she can discuss her treatment with tremendous clarity: 'I was telling the doctors at the meeting that five years ago I got a great deal better after having Anafranil drips, but I've been thinking about that since. I guess it wasn't the drips that helped mainly, so much as the psychotherapy that went along with it. Dr Brown saw me practically every day and spent a great deal of time talking to me and getting me deconditioned. And, you know, although he helped me over the particular obsession I had at that time there was this fear of germs as a subsidiary fear even then. I'd only been at home for two weeks when this began to take a hold of me!'

So Linda can explain what is wrong, in one sense. She has obsessional fears. What Linda cannot explain is why she has them. Maybe, when and if that is understood, Linda's 'illness' will be 'cured'. Meanwhile Linda might better be seen as having a problem she has to learn to live with. Or to use the words of a previous section, maybe Linda should be seen as having a disability that we all hope will not prove to be too great a handicap.

Whatever the terms we use, it may not be possible to resolve all the difficulties of the condition. The very best we may be able to do is to reduce the difficulties to a level where the patients can live tolerably.

And perhaps even most important of all, maybe we can initially accept the patients as likeable and understandable people as they are, and help their relatives and acquaintances to accept them as they are, and help the patients themselves to accept and to like themselves as they are. Not with a view to their staying that way for ever, but in the belief that from such a point they may go on to become the people they would better like to be.

Respecting the Patients' Choice

Five years before I ever began psychiatric nursing I copied this into my quotation book:

Problems are a dangerous hybrid of modern times. They seem to be meant only and solely to be talked about. How often you find when you earnestly try to help somebody with his problems, how often you learn to your own astonishment that he doesn't really want that. He needs problems in order to be able to talk about himself. This is a disease of our time. Just watch little children; they never have problems. They may have obstacles to encounter, and no-one is as persistent as a little child in trying to overcome an obstacle! They may have, small as they are, a cross to carry, and it is very touching to watch how patiently children suffer. But in their life is no room for a problem. They are not yet busy with themselves. (Trapp, 1956)

I introduced this topic very near the start of this book under the heading 'Me-me-me'. And I repeat here what I also said there: that we should not judge people for being turned in on themselves. It is an unenviable state.

From such experience as I have had, and I know it is not yet a very great deal, I feel strongly that many patients who might be helped, in fact dare not be helped. I can understand that, although I find it distressing and exasperating! It seems to the outsider, to the onlooker, to the nurses and others, as if their illnesses, their problems, their whatever we choose to call them, are a form of escape from lives they cannot cope with. When we say, 'We could help you', we appear to be offering to lead them back to those lives. And though many are glad to be helped, others dare not be.

The very first person to appear in this book was Stuart. A year ago - and, note well, *before* his complaint that we give too little attention to the fact that he and other patients worry about how long they are going to be here - he was offered a chance to live in a small home. To us it seemed an ideal and rare opportunity, but the prospect completely unhinged him. It was only with the greatest of reassurance and encouragement and support that he even went to see the home and meet the people who ran it. To the amazement of the kindly, mature student nurse who accompanied him, but not at all to the surprise of the social worker who also went, who knew such situations in general and Stuart in particular, Stuart gave an outstanding display of himself as grossly psychotic. Almost inevitably he was not even considered for a trial period in the home. And, of course, to our chagrin, the home must have doubted our sanity in recommending him!

Changing one's course of life takes courage for most people. For psychiatric patients it takes even greater courage. Their lives may at present be full of distress, but the distress is familiar. The unknown may seem worse.

I am writing especially with the longer-stay hospital patients in mind. The hospital has offered them a retreat from a world they could not cope with. And while they have been in hospital the difficult world outside has changed and has become even more difficult!

When all is said and done, we can do little unless the patients themselves do not want and dare to solve these problems.

And we will not get far in solving patients' problems if they themselves do not want and dare to solve those problems.

References

Mackarness, R. (1976). *Not All In The Mind*, London: Pan Books.

Trapp, M.A. (1956). *Yesterday, and Today, and Forever*, London: Geoffrey Bles.

Part Two:
The Viewpoint of the Staff

6 A Good Look at the Staff

In my early plans for this book, the staff had not only a chapter, but they had the first chapter! Called 'Happy staff in a happy hospital', its theme was that until the hospital staff's own morale is good, they cannot begin to help the patients. It owed its primary position to a bad patch of low morale that I was then working through myself, but once I was through it I was able to go back to 'Patients first', which has the job in much better perspective.

But from that low morale I learnt this lesson: that during such periods our perspectives are altered. Too much of our thinking, talking and concern is diverted to ourselves. We become like the patients: too 'me-me-me-ish'. If our morale becomes too low, there is nothing to distinguish us from our patients: we have a depressive illness, even including suicidal or paranoid thinking. We may become as withdrawn and disorganised as the schizophrenics, or drink as much as the alcoholics. On days when the work has gone well we may swing unnaturally high, only to swing back low again. And what of our patients then? Remember the old saying: 'Physician, heal thyself.' Paraphrase it: 'Psychiatric nurses should solve their own problems!'

This chapter will look at the staff, some of the problems, and some of the solutions.

Who Are the Staff in Psychiatric Hospitals?

In my first-line management course I was taught so-called 'brainstorming techniques', and am applying it here to get as complete a list as I can of all the staff who may be found in a psychiatric hospital. In random order, just as they come, they are:

Nurses	Laundry staff
Doctors	Sewing room staff
Porters	Path. lab. technicians
Electricians	Social workers
Carpenters	Ward clerks
Painters	Dentists
Occupational therapists	Hostel wardens
Industrial therapists	Librarians
Physiotherapists	Tutors
Domestics	Pharmacists
Radiographers	Catering staff
Voluntary workers	Cooks
Drivers	Restaurant staff
Secretaries	Accounts department staff
Research department staff	Medical records staff
Chiropodists	Legal experts
Administrators	Bank staff
Psychologists	Gardeners
Telephonists	Optician
Shop assistants	Art therapist
Hairdressers	Patients' teacher
Beauticians	Chaplains
Storesmen	

Let's leave them mixed up. The staff do not exist in tight compartments. They are involved with one another, and they all exist, directly or indirectly, to help the patients. They all need - to use another term which is becoming a cliché - job satisfaction. They need to feel of use, appreciated, and able to get on happily with their work without thinking, talking and worrying about it in an out-of-perspective way.

Fifty Niggles Felt by Staff at Work

It is so difficult to write about problems with colleagues, fellow-staff and friends, and the whole subject raises a number of points and questions:

First, maybe it is best to deal with this whole subject lightly. I for one could sink quite low merely by contem-

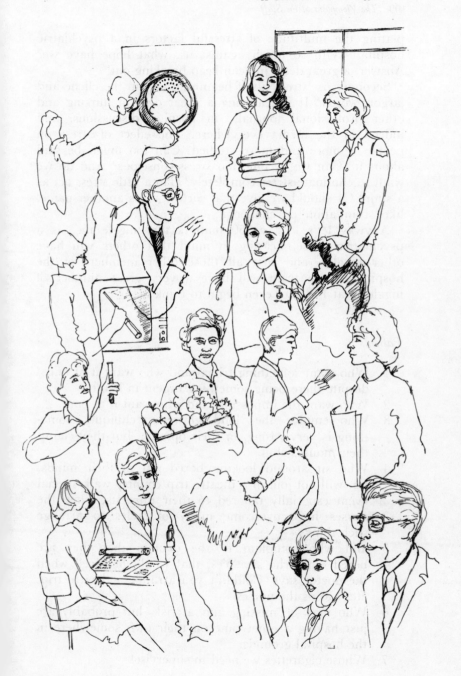

plating the multitude of stressful factors in a psychiatric hospital! With so much against us, what hope have we? Answer: a great deal. Joy can keep breaking out!

Secondly, is 'stress' itself beginning to join the cliché and jargon words? It is featuring a great deal in nursing and other professional journals, in hospital discussions, and indeed in the media everywhere. The effect of stress on people is more and more studied. Can too much be said about it? Can we become too stress-conscious? And do we want to eliminate stress completely? Can a little stress act as a spur? Or should we give that sort of stress another name, like 'stimulation' or 'challenge'?

Anyway let's look at 50 matters that niggle me, as a psychiatric nurse, bearing in mind that others will have other niggles, and that all those other members of the hospital's huge team will have a very great number of niggles that I cannot even begin to think of.

Patients

1   Who want something trivial and who want it at once, despite there being something urgent in hand.
2   Who want the impossible and who want it at once.
3   Who employ the 'loud glower' technique. Something is very wrong, in their opinion, but they clamp their mouths shut.
4   Who sit around looking bored out of their minds, but will not join in a theatre trip/country walk/special event especially tailored to their interests, when the nurses have overcome many obstacles to arrange such things -
5   and who complain to the doctors that they are bored, and who say 'Yes, that would be nice!' when the doctor says 'Couldn't you arrange a theatre trip, etc.?' to us the nurses!
6   Who may be missing and at risk, but probably are just having a quiet time on their own somewhere in the hospital grounds.
7   Whose cigarettes we need to supervise!

8 Who constantly home in on the staff whenever we have to talk to someone else - a relative, a tutor, or a social worker.

9 Who are helped into neatness and tidiness and who are back to their incredibly awful norm before the nurse can bat an eyelid.

10 Who are spiteful to a fellow-patient.

11 Who are young, obviously ill, yet unhelpable.

12 Who are young, not obviously ill, yet determined to be in hospital.

13 Who are jackdaws, to whose bed-area the nurse and patient have to take a rubbish bag, a laundry bag, bucket and water, and a tranquil mind. The last is hard to hang on to once the locker and drawers are opened!

14 Whose enjoyment appears to come from setting, for example, the nurses against one another.

Things that conspire against psychiatric nurses trying to do their job

15 Being unable to walk on one errand from A to B without seeing ten other jobs *en route*.

16 Having to put in a second or third order for something already dealt with.

17 Having to wait for days, weeks or even months for things which are needed now or very shortly.

18 Things that have gone missing.

19 Things that aren't working properly.

20 Forms to be filled.

21 Being given a fish tank and money for the fish, but not being allowed to have a water-heater or aerator because of some silly rule.

22 The phone, when it keeps ringing.

23 Lack of sufficient continuity, so that something begun by one person is inadvertently overlooked by the next.

24 Shortages of food, money, laundry, clothes.

Niggles related to hospital and ward managers such as nursing officers

25 Who come with all the complaints without balancing it by appropriate approval.

26 Who move staff too frequently.

27 Who have too many bright ideas for their staff to put into action!

28 Who invite the Top Brass to our ward events as showmanship.

29 Who have a basic psychiatry philosophy too different from my own.

30 Who don't keep their nurses enough in the picture.

31 Who overcommunicate, chiefly with memos which one ceases to read properly.

32 Who would have us at their meetings, discussions, lectures, courses, without realising that they are not the only arrangers of meetings, discussions, etc.

33 Who change their own complex plans too often.

34 Who use my ward office as a place where they can have a break from their stresses at a time when I have things I should love to get on with!

Others who niggle

35 Student nurses who are bored on the ward.

36 Student nurses who criticise too readily and who think we are fools.

37 Students who produce as a bright idea something we've been trying to achieve for years.

38 Student nurses who seem to hope we will do for them the work that their teachers have allocated to them to do.

39 The good nursing tutor who is dead-keen, but who chooses the wrong moment to try to stimulate us.

40 The 'jargon-ites' who talk dynamically of the latest idea as, if we have only to introduce this for total cures all round.

41 The 'below-par domestic'.

42 The member of another department who general-
   ises about 'nurses' as if we are a different species
   and all alike.
43 The patient's relatives who say 'Where's mother's
   teeth/specs/slippers?'
44 The relatives who think we fail by not producing a
   miracle cure.

Last straws

45 Moaners
46 Nurses who snipe about the opposite shift of nurses.
47 Speculators and rumour-mongers.
48 The over-tough ('What those patients need is
   firmness.')
49 The inflexible.
50 The lazy.

Following such a list, there are two other things I must say
at once: that I am never oppressed by all 50 difficulties at
once, of course, and that I have a basically bouncy nature,
and *can* overcome any one of them.

And what have my niggles and my nature to do with
you? I tell them only to make this point: that it seems to me
to be of paramount importance to have some self-
understanding, whoever we are, and especially if we work
in a psychiatric hospital. Just as a psychoanalyst must first
undergo psychoanalysis, so psychiatric nurses and others
working in psychiatric hospitals should know quite a lot
about themselves. But from experience, I suspect that
most of us do not look much at ourselves, either critically
or compassionately, nor do we look compassionately at our
colleagues.

The great danger in not doing so is that our reaction to
stress will be to hit out at others, with criticism, sarcasm,
envy, resentment or other destructive attitudes. And the
others in turn will pass this on. This is true for all those
who live and work in the psychiatric hospital, and not just
the nurses and other professionals. Sooner or later the

patients will also be affected by this chain of reactions, and they were stumbling to start with; that is why they are in the hospital. Our very job is to arrest their fall and to help them to stand upright!

Coming to Terms With Stress

RECOGNISING THE SYMPTOMS

Interestingly, we may recognise that something is wrong even before we can identify what it is. This is obvious when we are looking at other people, but it is often true too of ourselves.

So, first, learn to recognise your own symptoms of stress. A feeling of being unable to cope? Not being able to get off to sleep at night, or waking far too early in the morning? Other symptoms usually come before those, such as: believing that everyone else is incompetent; becoming overtalkative or too withdrawn; having no energy and losing one's memory alarmingly; becoming easily irritated, or openly bad tempered. Which is really the more draining: the psychogeriatric ward with its rounds of dressing, washing and toileting; the acute psychiatric ward where one may spend large amounts of time just sitting and listening; or the long-stay ward with its apathetic patients? The nurses on the first are convinced they must be the more tired, and yet the student nurses on the second and third may be amazed at their loss of energy.

I have a now-amusing recollection of a moment when I thought my mind must be going.

'That woman in the dormitory,' I said, 'shall I take her some Complan in a . . . '. I could see the thing in my mind. A tall drinking vessel. I knew there was even a choice of words and I couldn't remember one!

' . . . cup?' I finished lamely.

'A large beakerful, please', said the sister, unsuspecting.

Or a tumbler, or simply a glass! No problem now!

IDENTIFYING AND SORTING THE STRESSES

Once we are aware that we are showing symptoms of stress, the next thing is to ask ourselves exactly what it is that is bugging us this time. Sometimes the answer may be obvious: a hurdle to be leapt in the next few days, such as a ward event that we particularly want to go well. Or maybe a fellow staff member is needling us unreasonably. Or the fault may lie very much in ourselves: a tendency to over-react to criticism, an inflexibility, a fearfulness about new ideas. Being honest with ourselves as we try to identify the cause of our lack of ease may require some courage - and even when we think we have the answer we may well be deceiving ourselves!

But let's assume that we have a pretty good idea as to what is wrong. How do we deal with it?

There is an old prayer:

> God grant me
> Serenity to accept the things I cannot change,
> Courage to change the things I can,
> And wisdom to know the difference.
>
> (Green and Gollancz, 1962)

So, let's look at our current problems, and decide whether there is anything at all to be done? It may need courage, involving tackling someone of whom we are a little afraid, and it may need a lot of tact. But those who work with psychiatric patients are supposed to be psychologically more skilled than average - aren't we!

A CARTOON APPROACH

A tutor once put a most helpful book into my hands: *Illuminative Incident Analysis* (Cortazzi and Roote, 1975). Its basic theme is that, faced with difficulties, it is often helpful actually to draw them out rather than talk about them in words.

I remember two applications of my own. The first picture once helped me to identify my own mixed feelings.

Merely drawing the pictures of myself, as a yo-yo, a roaring lion, a firing cannon, cheered me up, and my fellow-staff laughed first and then understood me better.

The second picture tried, more seriously, to identify my reason or reasons for not being wholly happy with my ward. Because I like gardening I used a garden to represent the ward. The flowers are the patients. The gardeners are the regular ward staff. Once I'd got the idea it appealed to me more and more. Flowers are living, growing, varied, and capable of giving much pleasure and comfort. Some are immediately noticeable. I could see our bright Gloriana as a sunflower. Others are unostentatious little rockery plants, really delightful once noticed, like Maggy, Annie, Hannah and Jean. All those were patients who kept a very low profile, and all different. All flowers may, however, need help from the gardeners to be at their best. And what do the gardeners need? Training, experience - but they also need water. And maybe that was what we were lacking for our garden: adequate refreshment. No, not booze, nor yet more cups of tea, but stimulation chiefly. And perhaps we also needed reassurance and encouragement, and people taking an interest.

That was only the first cartoon in that set. Four more followed, varying solutions to 'What does a gardener do if there is too little water?'

Try the cartoon approach sometimes on your own problems - just draw out a picture of the situation you find yourself in.

USING SOME ASSERTIVENESS

Various articles and letters about meekness, assertion and aggression appeared in the *Nursing Times* in the spring of 1979. The chief discussion then was about training nurses out of meek submission, out of being mere 'handmaidens to the doctors', and out of cowering before frightening ward sisters. More recently, I have heard of Radical Nurses Groups and of the formation of the Psychiatric Nurses Association. There are, I know, many nurses who feel that they are not allowed as positive a role as they would wish.

My own standpoint as a psychiatric nurse is somewhat different. I do feel that I have been given a great deal of opportunity to speak up for myself, and that I have taken it. What I have seen in other nurses (and sometimes in myself), and felt sorry about, were bursts of verbal aggressiveness. Yes, I have realised that such bursts of anger were almost always the result of feeling threatened or frustrated in some way.

I too approve of a proper assertiveness as being yet another example of the golden mean! It is a middle way between lying down and being trampled over and jumping up at once in a battling attitude.

Assertiveness consists of being reasonable and adult, putting one's points clearly, cheerfully and without too much emotion, standing one's ground if necessary, and just laughing gently at those who would try to manipulate us. Sometimes this is easier said than done, but we need to persist!

PUTTING OURSELVES IN THEIR SHOES

This metaphor of putting oneself in other people's shoes has been used over and over in this book, and used unashamedly. I find it a helpful picture. Try to forget yourself. Imagine you really are that other person. Apply all that you know about them - and a hospital's gossippiness can actually be applied usefully at times: you may not have wanted to know about X's wife, Y's child, or Z's mother, but it may explain a little why they are not always sweet and reasonable every moment. Yes of course the perfectionists will argue that true professionals never bring their problems to work, and I would support them and say that the patients must come first and that our private lives must not intrude too much. But we are whole people, not just nurses or electricians or domestics or telephonists or shop assistants, and we must recognise each other as whole people.

But I am not advocating a nosey investigation into each other's out-of-hospital lives! I'm really asking us to step into each other's at-work role. It was such an eye-opener becoming a psychiatric ward sister! I really had thought, as a student nurse, that many of the sisters and charge nurses sat around in the office and did very little. And one of my own nursing assistants, a very likely lad, cheerful and chirpy and ideal both for our patients and as a fellow staff member, once shattered me by saying 'Well, there's not all that much to being a sister, is there! Just taking and sending telephone messages.' And he meant it!

And if we cannot step into the shoes of those so close to us, what hope have we of imagining the pressures on some of the others: the drivers, the psychologists, the bank staff and maybe also the psychiatric patients themselves.

But if we are already getting our attitudes to our patients right, we can apply those same attitudes to our fellow staff! Let's see them as people we work *with*, and treat them as basically normal and reasonable people, and try to understand why they sometimes are less reasonable than we would like, and recognise our own failings and the others' virtues a little more, instead of our own virtues and the others' failings! This may sound like simplistic preaching, and I can only say that when relating to one another is so important, and it is vitally important that the staff should do so, they cannot afford to wait until they are all fully qualified in psychology and psychological approaches. With problems between staff we have to start somewhere, and the use of our imaginations to help us put ourselves in one another's shoes is one of the best starting points of all!

Who are you, and who do you meet in the course of your work? Below is a random list of people in psychiatric hospitals. Start by being yourself and imagine the joys and frustrations of the work of each of those others. Not just any domestic, but your own Janet! Not just any head porter, but your own Mac! And then try it the other way on. Imagine you are Jim, the Senior Nursing Office or Pat who works in Industrial Therapy. How do you and how does your work look through their eyes?

Pharmacist

Chiropodist

Industrial therapy worker

Ward sister

Domestic

Head porter

Senior Nursing Officer

Sewing room woman

Paul Tournier (1962), a Swiss psychiatrist-cum-philosopher, puts the case for cooperation in place of competition as a lifestyle. I support that! One-upmanship as so brilliantly identified by Stephen Potter (1952) can be fun, as long as it is only a game. But what of those who are shoved down in the process when it is played for real?

LOOKING FORWARD

The older we get, the more nostalgic we become. At 50-plus I find myself talking occasionally about my parents' iron-framed mangle with wooden rollers that doubled as a scullery table!

As a student nurse one of my hardest trials was having to listen to 'It's not like it used to be.' The oldest nurses even sentimentalised about having to carry coal each morning to light the ward fires, and comparatively young ones recalled happy days working alongside the patients at 'bumping', which involved polishing the old wooden floors.

I wrote earlier about how hard it is to notice changes when we are in the middle of them. Hospitals are changing all the time. It is possible to make it sound as if our work is getting very much easier: the development of new tranquillisers, the introduction of domestic and of occupational therapy staff, the reduction of hours, student nurses being seen as learners and not as 'pairs of hands'.

The changes are many and rapid. Let us take three examples alone:

When I started my psychiatric nursing eight years ago, in 1973, I saw wards full of elderly patients confined in 'geriatric chairs'. For the younger nurses I must now explain that these had a table from chair arm to chair arm, and secured the man or woman into the seat. They were used with the best of intentions: to prevent the tottering and dementing patients from moving around restlessly and overactively, and falling and breaking limbs.

Again, at that time it was still the ward sisters and charge nurses of my training hospital who went out to visit ex-patients in their homes to give the depot injections. The Community Psychiatric Nurse was as yet almost unknown.

And our uniforms, yes, as psychiatric nurses, included starched white aprons. Oh, but here I am getting on to dangerous grounds. In my present hospital I have never had a uniform at all, but at my previous hospital my ex-colleagues are still in theirs. And perhaps some of them still regret the passing of their white apron that made them feel 'a proper nurse'.

Let's learn to let the past go, to grasp the good things of the present. I would count the improving staff-patient attitudes, the growing multidisciplinary approach, and the recognition of there being a social as well as a medical model in psychiatric care as high among our present virtues - and let's look forward to yet more good future developments. For myself, I can see that we are on the verge of learning a great deal more about helping patients to come to terms with themselves and their lives.

The future can be frightening to those of us who are growing older, who have struggled hard to get such qualifications as we have and who had thought we had got somewhere! But our hospitals are not going to stand still because we should like them to, so we had better accept our need to keep pace cheerfully!

It isn't easy. It is frightening. It takes a lot of honesty and laughing at ourselves. We must recognise that it is all right to say ... 'Help! I don't know anything about this. Tell me.' But it takes courage.

It took courage to let those tottery old folk out of their geriatric chairs. 'They'll all fall down and break their hips and then what will their relatives say? We'll be blamed and rightly so.' But they didn't all fall down. No more hips were broken than formerly were. Possibly less, as more of them kept the use of their legs.

The future can hold fresh delights for us, if we'll let it - but I want to add this:

Sheerly writing and thinking about this book has helped me to see things more clearly. I do very often feel overwhelmed and helpless in my work as a psychiatric nurse. It is frightening to feel I cannot cope as the ward sister, when others have coped before me and appear to be coping around me. But articles such as 'Voice of the ward sister' (Fairbrother, 1981) confirm our difficulties:

> The many other disciplines involved in ward life (one survey showed that on average a ward sister was interrupted no less than 64 times in the course of her shift) place a great strain on her 'specialist' role. Yet this role becomes even more important as other specialist roles increase. Having the ward at your fingertips is quite a challlenge these days, when plenty of other peoples' fingers are in the pie as well!

So I'm not just imagining that there's more to the job of a psychiatric ward sister than a bit of telephoning! And as long as other people understand that it is complex I can actually enjoy its complexities, for it is certainly not dull! But the main point of that article was that the work of a psychiatric nurse is changing, and that it is good for it to change.

LOOKING FOR JOY

A few lines of William Blake are now part of my personal

creed:

> Life is made of joy and woe
> And when this we surely know
> Through the world we safely go.

Anyone working in a psychiatric hospital who thinks that the job has no woes must be a very strange person indeed. But what sad people they are who have lost their awareness of the joys of working and living with psychiatric patients. There are dozens of joys, day by day. However, just sometimes they do have to be consciously looked for.

It was a tremendous joy lately noticing that Jean and Muriel were sitting at opposite ends of one of our small dining tables one supper time, eye to eye.

Me   Would you like a second supper, Muriel?
Muriel   That cornish pasty was good. Yes, I would like another. Unless Jean would like it.
Jean   No, it's all right. You have it, Muriel.
Me   There are two spare. You can each have one.
Jean and Muriel   Oh, thank you, sister!

Now that would be good, anyway. Different from the 'me-me-me stance' of which I wrote early in the book. But coming from those two! Unbelievable. Almost ludicrous. Their enmity had been so great. In one tussle, six months ago, Jean had banged Muriel's head against a washbasin and caused a nasty bruise. And yet, even on that occasion I suspected that she might have been provoked by Muriel's malice. But Jean herself can be extraordinarily foul-mouthed and frightening. She is a huge woman and when she scowls the whole ward feels apprehensive. Six weeks ago Muriel raised the matter of Jean's behaviour in a ward meeting (in Jean's absence, needless to say) and the ward was unanimous in asking that she might be specially seen by the consultant about her behaviour - and now!

I laughed at them both, gently and individually at first, but then we later laughed about it all together.

Jean, a very lonely but very warm-hearted woman, agreed that it was proving best to try to be nice to people because then they are nicer to you. Muriel did say, ominously, behind Jean's back. 'It won't last, of course. She won't be able to keep it up. There'll be trouble again, you'll see.'

But for the moment it is one of the joys!

GETTING AWAY FROM IT

I once hated those women's magazines' articles about people who were stars - film stars and good cooks; prima ballerinas and superb mothers; olympic athletes and talented painters. It was too much! Quite unfair when most of us weren't even starlets at anything!

But psychiatric nurses (and probably all nurses, and anyone in a job that can be stressful) will be better at their job if there are are few 'ands'! 'Let yourself off the hook just once in a while', says a song I like. I listen to a lot of music and belong to a Recorded Music Club, where I can share this pleasure with others. I love the countryside and have joined the Ramblers. I'm lucky in having married sons who come to stay with me with their wives, or who welcome me to them. I'm to be a grandmother for the first time this year!

What do you do out of work hours? There is sometimes a danger that psychiatric nurses will only meet other nurses and talk nursing? Don't - well, hardly ever!

The golden mean applies yet again! Get the balance right. And do get away, right away, as often as you reasonably can.

Go placidly amid the noise and haste, and remember what peace there may be in silence . . . Beyond a wholesome discipline, be gentle with yourself. You are a child of the universe, no less than the trees and the stars; you have a right to be here . . . With all its sham, drudgery and broken dreams it is still a beautiful world. Be careful. Strive to be happy.

Desiderata

References

Blake, W. (1757-1827). *Auguries of Innocence*.

Cortazzi, D. and Roote, S. (1975) *Illuminative Incident Analysis*, London: McGraw-Hill.

Fairbrother, C. (1981). 'Voice of the ward sister', *Nursing Focus*, March.

Greene, B. and Gollancz, V. (1962). *God of a Hundred Names*, London: Gollancz.

Potter, S. (1952). *One Upmanship*, London: Hart-Davis.

Tournier, P. (1962). *Escape from Loneliness*, London: SCM Press.

Part Three:

Looking at the Relatives of Psychiatric Patients

7 Relatives and Friends

Finding the Relatives

It is frequently a shock to outsiders to learn how long many patients have been in a psychiatric hospital. In the general hospital a patient will probably stay for ten days or so. In the psychiatric hospital, even today, there are patients still in their twenties who have spent most of the past ten years in the hospital. When our terrible, and somewhat simple, Meg was to have a minor gynaecological operation I rang the surgical ward sister first.

Me She can be very difficult, but I think you will have little trouble. She loves new experiences.
She What is her diagnosis?
Me It has varied over the years.
She Has she been in hospital long, then?
Me She's sixty now, and she came in at eighteen.
She (immediately pro-Meg) Oh, the poor thing! How awful!

And I was able to explain that, surprisingly, Meg's life in hospital had not been as awful as all that. But that is not the point here.

None of Meg's relatives had visited within anyone's memory. Yet Meg came from a large family. She had trotted out the names of all her seven siblings one relaxed afternoon and had told me much about them. I had amused Meg by drawing a sheet of pin-men and pin-women of them all (and had kept it for reference in her notes).

So few of our 30 patients were visited. We had a campaign to find the missing relatives. My letter to Meg's sister who was listed as her next-of-kin was returned with 'Not known at this address'.

Nora's sister had a very grand address. I guessed that she worked at 'the big house'. Now, decades later, she was probably untraceable. Marvels, she had moved to a cottage in the same small village.

One moving reply came from a son-in-law. 'I am sorry to tell you that my wife died some years ago. I never met my mother-in-law, but I shall be happy to do anything I can.'

A contrasting reply from old Annie's niece and nephew-in-law: 'We see no point in visiting her. We have had little contact for many years.' Yet they came the very same day when she was seriously ill. They seemed a nice couple. As well as welcoming them and making it easy for them to talk with Annie, I took them to her work area. The staff greeted them with joy and were full of praise for Annie. It was clearly an eye-opener for them that their 'strange' relative commanded such respect. This story had a sequel which was incredible to me: when Annie recovered, they still would not visit her despite my further invitations.

Getting the Relatives to Come

Putting ourselves into the relatives' shoes, we could see that a visit to a 'lunatic asylum', as it was probably still seen, or even to a psychiatric hospital, could be a difficult experience, involving apprehension in advance, anxiety and tension on the occasion, and a great mixture of feelings in retrospect. The long-stay wards of a psychiatric hospital never normally see the droves of visitors which are characteristic of visiting time in a general hospital, and there is no doubt at all that the single visitor does get stared at, especially on the first appearance. Consider the patient's point of view: 'Who is this? I've never seen this person before. Oh, she's come to see Bertha. Fancy! Is it her sister? What's she come for?' The deeply introverted patient may squint sideways repeatedly at the visitor. The paranoid patient may glower unwaveringly. The manic may rush up! 'Who are you? What have you come for? I'm Doris. I have a sister, too. She lives in Birmingham ... ' until a nurse leads her away, cross and protesting.

We decided to have a party. The few relatives who normally came singly could meet, and their presence would make it easier for the strangers. That very presence would say, even without the words, though no doubt some would actually be spelling it out: 'We too have the burden and anxiety of a mentally ill relative.'

The invitations went out with PTO on the front, and an appropriate personal message on the back. Each situation was individual, remember! We had no idea whether our first get-together would be a success or a gigantic flop. But the RSVP's brought responses, and the day brought the visitors.

Nora's sister had written 'I am sorry it is so many years since I came. Nora is my only sister and was very dear to me. May I bring a friend with me?' They were the first to come. Guilt and remorse and promises: 'I feel terrible. Whatever must Nora think of me! I'll make it up to her. I'll come every month without fail.'

My first inward reaction: 'Oh yeah? We'll see, shall we?' And she could have slipped back again, but with a little friendly chivvying the relationship was renewed and stayed strong until Nora's death.

Nora's first reaction? Joy? Sulks? Neither. She just did not have a clue who this stranger was.

'My sister? Oh, hullo, me old duck.'

We were all 'me old duck' to Nora. The stranger meant very little to her at first.

Obviously I must summarise. From this first gathering on the ward we went on to others. A Christmas party with carols, and the discovery of the talents of some relatives at singing and playing. A get-together out of the hospital, when we took most of the patients (some were unbudgeable and we reluctantly allowed them to be so) by coach to a great park, where the relatives met us and carried off their mothers, aunts, sisters, daughters and wives to explore its various attractions until we re-met for a high tea in the restaurant.

And, for those readers who I hope are wondering about this: for those who had no relatives we invited relative-substitutes to our gatherings. Some were staff of the occupational and industrial therapy units in the hospital, others were regular volunteers, the hospital hairdressers, the tea-room ladies: many of them people who did not normally come much to the ward. 'Come and see us in our "home" setting', we said on that first occasion. And with only a minimum of prompting they 'adopted' the relativeless patients for the event, while other patients were drawn into their friends' family groups.

Involving Relatives and Friends

Two years after our first relatives' gathering, ten of our ward's 30 patients were planning to go on a week's summer holiday and we needed to raise funds. Our efforts included an old-fashioned concert. It was great! Romantic ballads by Doris's brother-in-law and Lizzie's daughter. A Palm Court Trio with a former student nurse on her cello and two of her outside friends. Comedy turns from Gill, the occupational therapy aide who was to join us on the holiday. Community singing with Maureen's brother-in-law at the piano.

The holiday was in a seaside town where some of the relatives lived. 'Will it be possible for Mum to come to tea on Tuesday?' said Lizzie's daughter. And then 'That was marvellous! An old neighbour of hers came round. You should have heard them swopping stories! Would you let her come for the day on Thursday and then stay the night too?'

'Let her!' As if we were doing the relatives a favour!

'Can Nora come to my little cottage one day while you're so near? I'd love her to see it', said her sister.

The relatives came with us on a coach trip and on a boat trip. By the end of the holiday our roles had become very blurred. Patients? Relatives? Nurses? We were Nora, Vera, Margaret, May, Daphne, Linda, Gill, . . . Who was helping who?

The Invaluable Triangle

Relatives, staff, patients, if properly involved, form an invaluable triangle. Of course, if one has to pick out one as more important than another it must be the patient, who is the sole cause for the psychiatric hospital and those of us who work in it. But it is almost impossible properly to express the support that each can give the other.

Staff-patient is obvious and gets taken for granted. But the very purpose of this *New Approaches to Care* series of books is to help us re-look at the help we must give our patients.

Patient-staff links: the honest nurse will acknowledge the raised morale she gets from a patient's genuine appreciation, however expressed.

Staff-relative and relative-staff relationships: already the support that these can give each other will be becoming clear. I will expand this further shortly.

Relative-patient and patient-relative links: there is a saying: 'God gave us our relations. Thank goodness we can choose our friends!' And there is truth in this. But there is truth also in the belief that there's no-one quite like 'our ain folk', the family, the people who are 'ours' and to whom we 'belong'. As long, that is, as this is a mixture of mutual caring and sharing, and not a devouring possessiveness.

Accepting the Relatives

Ultimately, when we really know the relatives, we shall find ourselves accepting them 'warts and all' in just the same way as the best nurse begins to accept her colleagues and patients. This involves recognising that they are human beings too, like ourselves. Recognising that though they have their failings, they also have their strengths, and their needs.

But first we have to accept them on a much simpler level. I cannot have been the only student nurse who was advised by some ward staff to 'Be careful of the relatives. They can stir up so much trouble.' We may look at the relatives with suspicion, as if they are enemies. It is the 'Here is a stranger, heave a brick at him' approach.

Quite often we have a dislike, which we may or may not acknowledge, which comes from a possessiveness we have developed. Here is Mr Smith making very clear that *our* Bertha is *his* mother!

On the acute wards especially, the nursing staff's attitude to the relatives may be quite complicated, and we may need to ask ourselves what it is we are feeling and why. As a wife whose marriage was crumbling I was entirely sympathetic towards one depressed wife: 'Poor woman! What an unimaginative husband she has! What little affection he gives her! Sister says he is very concerned . . . Poppycock!'

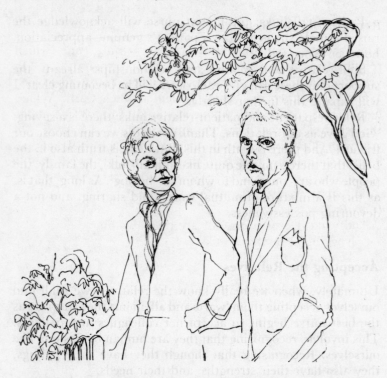

We are in fact taught that few psychiatric patients have become 'ill' in total isolation. That even if there is a physical cause to their illness, there are probably environmental and psychological causes too. 'Look at the relatives' we are told. And we do: 'Have you met Rosina's mother?' we ask one another . . . 'You can see why Rosina's as she is!' And maybe that is true, though I believe we are often too glib with such comments and far too judgemental.

Where is the buck to stop? What made Rosina's mother the way she is? Her parents? And what made them the way they were? Don't we get right back to Adam?

Let's accept this as quite likely: that much of the way we are is because of our parents and our upbringing. Now what?

The patients on the long-stay wards may have very few relatives with whom they are in touch. As nurses, let's be sure we are not contributing to scaring off the relatives when they first come.

Recognising the Relatives' Needs

This section could be framed like a quiz; one which requires you to be specific. You cannot respond . . . 'Oh yes, I've certainly met relatives like that.' You need to ask: Who? Which relative? Which patient? Which ward? Which home? This section isn't about any kind of needs; it's about the relatives' needs. Like Pauline's mother who says, 'Oh yes, we get on fine when she comes home for weekends, as long as she has her own way in everything.'

So, what relative have you met who:
Is constantly giving way?
  And what degree of trouble are they avoiding:
    Nagging? Whining? Sulks?
    Temper tantrums?
    Broken property?
    A physical attack?
Is frightened that the illness may recur in another member of the family?
  In himself/herself?
  In someone who at present is a child?
  With reason?
  Because they know too little about psychiatric illness?
Feels guilty?
  Because they feel they should be looking after the patient themselves?
  Because they feel they may be partly/largely to blame for the patient's illness?
  Because they often feel hostile towards the patient?
Feels hostile to the patient or to the staff?
  Because they too often have to give way?
  Because they are afraid/feel guilty?
  (Yes, some of these do go round in circles! In this connection it is well worth reading *Knots* (Laing, 1970).)
  Because they feel too little is being done to make the patient better?
  Because they feel the patient is being neglected?
Is resentful?
  Because their lives are suddenly and unexpectedly

unable to continue as they had thought they would?
Because for years they have not had a 'normal' life?
Is afraid they will be 'saddled' at home with a very difficult
    person?
With a parent who has now become childish and
    child-like?
With a 'grown-up' son/daughter who has not grown up
    emotionally or responsibly, though in intelligence they
    may be perfectly able?
With a brother or sister who has spent years in a hospital
    and who is now also suffering from the effects of
    institutionalisation?
Is absolutely bewildered?
By the growing dementia of an elderly husband/wife?
By a sudden acute illness of a young husband/wife/son/
    daughter?
By behaviour they cannot understand, and by its going
    on and on without any obvious hope of a cure?
Is persistent that something surely might be done some-
    where by someone?

For the relatives' sake I should like to think you had not
met such folk. But if you haven't, it is simply because you
have not yet come across them or listened to them well
enough.

Helping the Relatives

One of my chief points in this book is the individuality of the
work involved in caring for psychiatric patients. It is so difficult
and so unwise to generalise. On each occasion we need to
respond to this particular person in this particular situation.
    Ian can look very strange at times. A short, slim young man
in his late twenties he experimented with drugs at university
and has since spent most of his life as a solitary, deluded and
hallucinating schizophrenic given to extremely noisy outbursts
which occasionally include threats of violence to himself or to
his parents. And having written that summary I at once need to
hedge it around with questions, qualifying comments and

disclaimers. Did the drug-taking cause the illness, or was it a symptom of an illness that was already there? He is one of the most 'schizophrenic' of our patients, but we still ask ourselves 'Is this primarily a genetic "illness", or has it chiefly psychological causes and should we be saying that Ian "has problems"?' How deluded is Ian? Does he really believe he has a pretty young wife called Jillie whom we keep from him, and a lavish apartment in New York? Or are these escapist fantasies that he often recognises himself to be no more than that? And although threatening in moments, we can allow him to go out into the town alone for a new record he has set his heart on without any anxiety.

Ian's parents form a near-perfect triangle with the hospital staff and with Ian. They talk freely to us, and we to them, and Ian is more often included in on the talking than not. We chat casually over matters that are in fact very important, standing at the door of the clinic room, perhaps, when his parents have collected the tablets for one of his twice-weekly spells at home. Ian is at home almost as much as he is in hospital. He himself finds both places necessary: the space of the hospital and the ready acceptance of the people here, many with problems like himself; and the small, normal, comfortable home that is his own, and to which the family's visitors come as usual.

That too is very much part of the help for Ian: that he is included in on so much that is normal.

'I admire you for that', I told Ian's mother. 'How do you find your friends take Ian?'

'Fine now. It wasn't easy at first. At first we had to come to terms with everything ourselves. But once we were sure where we stood and what we felt, then we were able to allow others in on the difficulties. Mind you, we did ask ourselves whether it was fair on the people who weren't a part of the family at all. Would it distress them too much?'

'And hasn't it often been helpful to them to meet Ian? Helpful to see how much of a person - and a reasonable person - Ian still is?'

'Indeed it has! And of course, so many people have opened up about their own experiences. So many have a mentally ill relative and have not felt able to talk about it.'

Peter's new step-father had once been in a mental hospital

himself, he told us. Such a jolly, chirpy little man, he so small and Peter so large, he has done Peter so much good. A year ago Peter would have prevented his mother's re-marriage. Supporting Peter and supporting his mother through the weeks prior to the marriage had not been simple. Yet now the new man in Peter's life so often has put a twinkle on to Peter's sad face when they come back together from Peter's frequent home visits.

And Peter's new 'Dad' comes from the same Welsh town as Derek's father. They discovered it at our Christmas party. 'Do you remember that shop at the corner of Cardiff Road?' they were saying to each other. All this normal contact between relatives can help.

This has been a motley collection of paragraphs looking at the question 'How do we help the relatives?' Let's spell out the nearest we get to an answer:

> Know the patient as well as possible.
> Help them to feel at ease with you.
> Know the relatives as well as possible.
> Make them feel welcome.
> Let both the patient and the relatives know you.
> Listen, listen, listen.
> Respond both as yourself, and as the professional you are trained to be.

An example of the last: 'Oh dear, I feel sad enough myself about Ian - and I can walk away from it all at the end of a shift! I know how I'd feel if one of my sons were so troubled. However, the whole concept of schizophrenia is changing; there is a lot of re-thinking going on. There's an interesting man in the research department here I've met recently; he's very interested in family work. Shall I find out if it could be useful for Ian's parents to have a chat with him some time?'

But I wouldn't necessarily say that to Ian's parents. And to Peter's and to Derek's parents I'd be saying things I wouldn't be saying to Ian's!

Above all we must be honest, and as practical as possible - just two more examples.

In 1975 the BBC broadcast a taped journal of comments from a woman who was coping alone with a greatly demented mother for whom there was no room in a psychiatric hospital. *Where's the Key?* it was called. The piece I shall never forget showed her anger about the visits of the community nurses. She felt they came only to keep her going without the real help she needed.

Only two days ago I was surprised by the visit to the ward of Stephanie's mother. Her daughter has just been transferred to another ward. She said she had come to thank us for our help to Stephanie. I think she had come chiefly to thank us for our help to herself. She said several times how marvellous it had been that she had been able to talk as much as she had. And she singled out for praise the ward's registrar: 'He was very honest with me. I did not like all he said. But I could say all I wanted to in return. I knew where I stood with him. And he seemed an understanding man.' Like the others in the patient-staff-relative triangle, the relatives recognise it if we step into their difficult shoes, and show that we can understand.

References

Laing, R.D. (1970). *Knots*, London: Tavistock Publications.

Postscript:

Life Beyond the Psychiatric Hospital

8 Beyond the Hospital

Putting the Book in Perspective

It is time for a reminder about this book - remember it is
'one nurse's view' (my view), the view of someone whose
entire psychiatric career, apart from a few weeks in
training, has been within a psychiatric hospital.

The book so far has been about hospital-based patients,
and the hospital staff, and the relatives - the invaluable
triangle. We have been putting ourselves into the shoes of
each of these three groups in turn. Well, I have! And you
have too, probably. Those I have failed to convince will
have stopped reading by now, I imagine.

But patients do get out of hospital. This is a vital aim of
psychiatric care. Look back at the account of the ward
holiday at the end of Chapter 3. That holiday was very
hard work, even though it was enjoyable. It was not
attempted out of masochism, or showmanship, or as a useful exercise for student nurses. It was aimed at getting a
group of long-stay patients out of the hospital, initially for
a week, and then for ever if any could go on to that.

It is very well appreciated now that only part of
psychiatric care is within a hospital. I won't attempt an
exact proportioning of hospital to community care, but
much less than half is within a hospital. At first I thought
that this book on psychiatric nursing would have a large
section about the out-of-hospital patients. But as I have
written about the in-patient care the space available for the
out-patient aspect has shrunk almost to vanishing point. I
am aware of even more I would have liked to have said
about the in-patient work, and I can only quote a sentence
of Laing which has long comforted me: 'One cannot say
everything at once.'

The 'Get-Them-Out' Movement

It seems astonishing that I, who have been in psychiatric nursing for what seems so short a period, can remember a time without psychiatric nurses working in the community (CPNs). I was on my first ward, a late beginner, when the staff nurse, about the marry and move to another county, told us about the job she had been offered there: almost entirely out of hospital, chiefly visiting people in their own homes, with a car provided, and going just once a week to the hospital to report and to receive fresh instructions. This was, I believe, before any community training was available in the UK.

These days, the student psychiatric nurse of the 1980s will be familiar - or will very soon become familiar - with the work of the Community Psychiatric Nurse. There is so obviously a need for psychiatrically trained nurses to work outside the hospital, supporting those who are glad to live as normally as possible but aware of their need for help at times; supporting the other supporters - the relatives, landladies, neighbours, friends, and leaders of clubs to which the ex-patient goes; liaising with the local doctor and reporting back to the hospital-based consultant.

For some psychiatric nurses, especially for those who are newly arrived in the field, this get-them-out move has been exciting. It promised even more variety and interest in our work than we had first foreseen. But for some of those who were used to psychiatric work being securely within the psychiatric hospital it was disturbing. Sisters and charge nurses were increasingly spending time away from their wards to follow up their discharged patients. Some - and especially those who were onlookers and not participants - saw this as disruptive. Could the hospital afford to lose the time the community-visiting nurses would have been giving to the in-patients? Would everyone soon be expected to follow up their ex-patients, and what about those who did not drive? How great was the exodus of patients and staff to be? Was the time coming, and if so how soon, when all the work would be out of hospital? Certainly a consultant within my training hospital was predicting the closure of the hospital as we knew it within the working lives of even us older nurses. For some it was bothering and threatening.

That last paragraph was written, you will notice, in the shoes of the staff. But what of the patients?

The patients being discharged over that period fell into two main groups.

First, there were those for whom discharge was expected and accepted: those who had come recently when acutely ill and for whom a brief period in hospital was all that was needed - for the moment, anyway. They might go on shuttling between home and hospital, in and out, through our 'revolving door'. The only difference was that the newly developing depot injections were apparently getting people better more quickly and keeping them out for longer, or for always. There was going to be, so it then seemed, a running down of the long-stay wards as their old inhabitants died and were not replaced.

But secondly, and this provoked the greater comment, there was a movement to get people out of hospital even from the long-stay wards themselves! Some of those patients were also benefiting from the depot injections and, guaranteed at least a fortnight's stability at a time without the need to live from tablet to tablet three times a day, they could as well live outside the hospital as in. And some really were better anyway and no longer needed many tablets. The florid illness had faded over the years. So why were they in hospital? Why not out?

And so they were got out. This is not the book in which to describe in depth all the work that was involved. Let's just state that the patients went to group homes, where several former patients lived as a family together; or to sheltered accommodation, under the care of a kindly landlady, perhaps one who had formerly run a boarding house for short-stay visitors and who was happy to exchange her fluctuating unknown guests for a permanent 'family'. The preparation was immense: finding the accommodation and helping the neighbours to accept the idea of ex-psychiatric patients next door; re-training the long-stay patients to run their own home with all that that included; finding supportive landladies and helping them to understand what their new guests and their needs might be like; finding day-time occupation for those who would be living out of the hospital for the first time for decades.

The hard work for many hospital staff was not made easier by the cynicism from others or by the fear at times from the patients themselves. There were stories galore, some marvellous, some so sad: of the known suicides and attempted suicides; of the reported unkempt and un-cared-for. For myself I learnt to suspend judgement about 'Have you seen so-and-so lately? They got her out and now she wanders the street looking lost and unhappy!' Sometimes it probably was so; one could only hope that enough care was going into all this to ensure that most who left were going out to better lives. There certainly were plenty of stories like these:

Katie   You've no idea what it means to have your own front door key after all these years!

Betty (over a cup of coffee with a former nurse she has welcomed to her new home)   It's been lovely to see you! But did you hear about Mrs Jones coming! I didn't really want to invite her in, but it seemed a bit of an official visit. She looked all round and said how well we were doing, and then she said she'd like a cup of coffee - so I took her to the door and directed her to the nearest cafe! Naughty, I know, but I did enjoy it!

The patients' relatives were being told of their move outside. John had had two sisters. Where were they now? Persistent detective work and some apprehension traced them. Would they want to hear of the brother they'd not seen for 40 years. Their tears were tears of amazement and joy. They had been advised all those years ago that John could never improve and that it would be better for them to stay away and forget him. They included him and his new group home 'family' back into their own wide family circle.

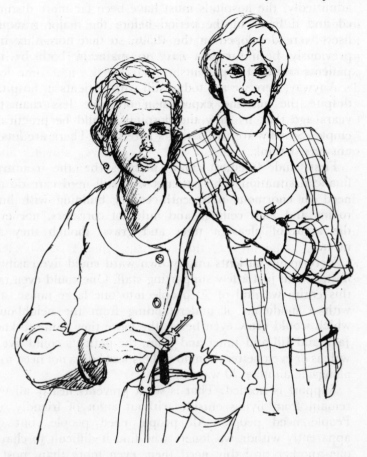

The move to get people out helped revolutionise the hospitals. Not only did the numbers of psychiatric patients in hospital drop by a third or more, but the very re-teaching of normal living to those who needed to re-learn it urgently for their new lives brushed off also on to those who were staying. A great awareness developed for normal living within the hospital and from the hospital-home.

This may be far too simplified. Maybe there had always been nurses who knew from instinct the importance of seeing and of stressing and encouraging the normal. And, admittedly, the hospitals must have been far more disturbed and difficult in the period before the major tranquillisers were developed in the 1950s, so that normality had previously been far less easy to maintain both by the patients and for the patients.

Anyway, here we are today still with patients in hospitals despite the genuine expectation of some less than ten years ago that by now the hospitals would be practically empty. So why are the patients here now? There are lots of answers, I think.

First and foremost may perhaps be the country's financial situation. The patients who still need care do not need an enormous nineteenth-century building with huge rooms and high ceilings and miles of corridors, nor even the acres of pleasant trees and grass, though they are nicer.

Very many patients on my own ward could live easily in hostels with just a few supporting staff. One could even take this entire wardful of 30 people into one large house, and with a modicum of understanding from the neighbours, which would grow even better the more they came to know Jack and Jill and Janet and John, the patients could live as well as or even better than now. This ward does not need to be alongside another 20 wards.

Support is needed. That is what prevents nearly all who remain from living outside without a lot of friendly aid. People need people. All people need people, but our apparently withdrawn loners who find it difficult to chat to one another probably need them even more than most of us. If our patients do have families - and not all do now have known relatives - the families have gone on without these members. It is unreasonable to expect brothers and sisters to open the doors of their present homes to include in a near-stranger they scarcely knew properly 20 or 30 years ago and to risk again the emotional upheavals to both the siblings and to the new household too. It is unreasonable even to expect parents to go on making a home for their child who has never developed emotional maturity and self-reliance.

This is a big subject which is emotional in itself. It is so easy for us nurses to say 'How awful of his parents not to want him! Look at the two of them in a nice home with a spare bedroom, when we are looking for somewhere to place their son! Ridiculous!' But is that really where it is best for Jack himself to be? Thirty years old, or more, unable to work, and still childish as well as child-like and especially so when on leave home to his parents.

No, what we also need are substitute families. Many many more hostels where people can develop into a caring, mutually supportive family. Or smaller groups, with or without substitute mums and dads or substitute brothers and sisters in the form of sympathetic and encouraging landladies and landlords. We haven't enough. Not nearly.

I wrote earlier, in 'Patients and diagnoses' of 'the grey area', of the patients who were neither obviously schizophrenic nor obviously psychopathic. That large group who, if anything, seem merely - yet tragically - inadequate. It is being, horrifyingly, realised that as our numbers of schizophrenic patients drop, being kept out of the hospitals with improved drugs and a much better approach to psychiatric illness and with the effort of rehabilitation, the hospitals are now almost being besieged by inadequate people who long for our support. This is why I wrote, very early in this book, that we might well, these days, revert to the term 'asylum'. A place of safety.

But then, we go round in circles. I have been saying in this section that most of our patients could live outside and do not need the hospital. One paragraph back I said we need substitute mums and dads and have too few. But now I recall a conversation with a Resettlement Officer whose express task was to find such accommodation. We were trying to find a home for Tim, aged 28, who within the hospital and without pressures was as normal as could be, but who had worn out a succession of substitute homes.

Me You'd think there'd be lots of women on their own who'd be glad to let a room to Tim and make some money and have him dropping in and out.

She (wide-eyed) You really think that? I wouldn't do it!

Me (wide-eyed in turn)   Oh, wouldn't you?

But on reflection, once I'd taken away my idealism, no, nor would I. I have come across too many Tims in psychiatric nursing. It's far too testing to have such a person permanently around me. I can cope with such people because at the end of my duty I can walk away.

A digression, and a question. When life is far, far too difficult, do the gentler folk who hate trouble retreat from the ordinary world into madness, and do the more determined stay in touch but keep on testing those around them? Could it be often as simple as this? And what part do genes play in both cases?

Anyway, a summary: the effort to get people out of hospital continues, but with great difficulty. For one reason and another many people need on-going support, and for one reason and another there are not yet enough alternatives to the large hospital.

The 'Keep-Them-Out' Movement

THE HOSPITAL AS A SUPPORT

I want to continue talking about psychiatric care in the community, and to describe a few of the ways our ward has contributed to the keep-them-out movement.

Once this was a rehabilitation ward. A great deal of effort went into teaching people to cook and sew, to use the phone, to handle money, and much more. But our present patients can do many of those things, passably, at least. Our main aim now is to create an atmosphere in which people can live as normally as possible, and from which people can leave when they wish to and when suitable accommodation outside is available.

We *also* want to create an atmosphere in which people can live as normally as possible and to which people can *come* when they need to! Over the past two years we have had a dozen or so community-based patients who have come to us for a very short while, only for the express purpose of taking a breather and coming to themselves again.

There is elderly Adeline, older in years than most of the patients on the ward, but so young in spirit. She lives alone in her country cottage for ten months of every year but comes in for December 'because it is a cold month and because it includes Christmas and it is nice to have company for Christmas' and for May 'because the spring flowers are over then and the raspberry crop has not started'. We are aware, as I am sure her neighbours and fellow villagers are aware, that Adeline has some strange beliefs. Sometimes the wonder is not that Adeline is permitted to use the hospital as she does ('Reason for admission?' asks the Medical Records Department twice a year and I am tempted to put down 'Because the spring flowers are over'!), but that Adeline survives in her somewhat lonely life outside for ten months of each year. It is our two months of care that help to keep her out for ten.

This year we have had Irene during her physical illness. Last year Irene had a spell with us while mentally ill. This year the prospect of a possibly serious operation was frightening, and Irene had no-one she knew well to talk to while she waited to be admitted to the general hospital. That was awful, she said. So she came in. I thought it good that we could help our former friend in this way. Our young staff nurse found it sad: 'I think it is dreadful that she hasn't anywhere else she can go except a psychiatric hospital.' Irene herself was content. And she helped the ward. She raised our reasonable level of normality further still, and she turned the other patients' thoughts away from themselves for a while. When Irene's operation at the local hospital was followed by a course of radiotherapy at a more distant hospital, the other patients were sad and concerned.

I could go on and on. There's Rosemary who rings up regularly from home for a chat and who stays here occasionally. And Pam who drops in for meals (don't tell our catering manager!) when she has blown all her invalidity money on bingo or on bookies.

It comes back to relationships again. A loose attachment to the hospital, an easy approachability to the in-hospital staff, may well be part of the keep-them-out movement.

And in this we are closely allied with the social workers and with the community psychiatric nurses. There is a great deal of easy relating and of flexibility between us too.

One important facility out there in the community is the 'tea and chat' club. What an awful name, I think! But it describes the club exactly. I have on my desk in connection with this book a long description of our nearest club (which has this name though others do not); of who founded it and who runs it; and also a hearty invitation to call in sometime. I shall indeed call, not as originally intended to gather material, but to meet ex-patients again in their out-of-hospital setting, and to meet again the helper who came from the club to the ward when one of her members was admitted for a short while.

All this brief section will do is bear tribute to those many groups, trained and untrained, from the highly organised and specialist Day Hospitals to the small voluntary clubs. There are very many more groups than those of us who work in psychiatric hospitals realise, and they make it possible for the lonely to come together at least occasionally. Their staff help with the prime task of keeping some sort of relationship going for those who find this difficult. And, in consequence, they help to keep ex-patients out of the psychiatric hospitals and others from ever becoming patients at all.

LOOKING TO THE FUTURE

A few pages back I described my interest nearly ten years ago in the newly starting work of psychiatric nursing in the community.

A few months ago one of my ward students was explaining that she hopes to be attached directly to a general practitioner. Some GPs, she said, are realising the value of having not just a general nurse linked to the practice, but a psychiatric nurse too. Yes. That makes sense. And very rewarding work it could be.

A few days ago a former student, now a staff nurse, told me about a visit she had lately made to a London centre where anyone can drop in and say 'I'm bothered. I think I need help. Things are getting on top of me.' Or whatever they want to say. And see psychiatrically trained nurses and consultants if needed, and social workers. And be steered in whatever direction is needed. Towards legal advice perhaps. Not necessarily towards psychiatric help at all. Whatever is needed can be given, informally at first, unofficially, and quickly, early. Before the beginning of a problem has ever turned into a mountain of a 'psychiatric illness'.

That's great, isn't it! How many more developments must be round the corner for the disturbed, lonely and psychiatrically ill. I can't wait for the future!!

Appendix:
Further Reading for Readers and Non-Readers

One of the main reasons why I insist that this book is largely my own view of psychiatric nursing is the amount I am not reading! The weekly nursing journals, the monthly nursing journals and the quarterly - I have indeed taken them, and I have watched them pile up unread, and I have grown depressed by my failure to be interested.

And then I found a passage in a book that cheered me. The book is *A Life of One's Own* (Field, J., Chatto and Windus, 1934. Also, Penguin, 1954). I came on it by chance in a second-hand bookshop. Joanna Field was the pseudonym of a psychologist who was trying to find out more about the way she herself ticked. She tells how for a long time she was continually putting off the next step in her exploration because she felt she ought to know more, and knew there were many books that she felt she ought to read before she could go any further. It took her years, she said, before she learnt that she must never begin her search by looking in books. She learnt to observe first, express what she observed, and then, if she needed it, see what the books had to say.

How that encouraged me! That was the way that I had been working.

But Joanna Field ended that passage by acknowledging her debt to books: 'Yet because I was daunted by the imposing array of printed information I must not minimize my debt to it. Probably reading has influenced my thought far more than I know.'

So here below is a small sample of books which have contributed greatly to my thinking, often by confirming what I have found for myself in my experience and by putting it into far better words than I could have done. These will not be your books, almost certainly. They are listed merely to show what a variety of books can influence us.

And if you do not want to read at present, so be it - especially if it is because you feel to be learning so much from what you are experiencing.

Fiction
Pym, B. (1958). *A Glass of Blessings*, London: Jonathan Cape.

Children's fiction
Jansson, T. (1948). *Finn Family Moomintroll*. (First published in English 1950, London: Ernest Benn.)

Biography
Russell, B. (1967). *The Autobiography of Bertrand Russell*, London: Allen and Unwin.

Poetry
Thomas, R.S. (1964). *Poetry for Supper*, London: Hart-Davis.

Letters
Hanff, H. (1971). *84 Charing Cross Road*, London: Deutsch.

Essays
Bacon, F. (1561-1626). *Essays*, especially 'Of Friendship'.

Allegory
Lewis, C.S. (1946). *The Great Divorce*, London: Geoffrey Bles.

Art
Escher, M.C. (1960). *The Graphic Work of M.C. Escher*, translated from the Dutch by John E. Brigham, Oldbourne Book Co. (Pan Books edition 1975).

Plays
Thomas, D. (1954). *Under Milk Wood*, London: J.M. Dent.

Psychotherapy
Rogers, C.R. (1967). *On Becoming a Person,* London: Constable.

Psychology
Peck, M.S. (1978). *The Road Less Travelled,* New York: Simon and Schuster.

Prayers
Kossoff, D. (1977). *You Have a Minute, Lord?* London: Robson Books.

Diaries
Kilvert, F. (1938-1940). *The Diary of the Rev. Francis Kilvert,* three vols, ed. William Plomer, London: Jonathan Cape.

Published talks
Priestland, G. (1981). *Yours Faithfully,* London: Fount Paperbacks, Collins.